In-Vitro Fertilization:
the Ultimate Reality Game

a true IVF story

Karen Daniels

In-Vitro Fertilization: The Ultimate Reality Game

DEDICATION

For Moms – wanna be and already there.
Keep moving forward. You're awesome.

ACKNOWLEDGMENTS

Thank you to my fellow PPSers
and other IVF journeyers,
brave women all.

To C – who was there from the beginning and held my
hand.

And to S.G.B. for support and editing -
in all areas of my life.

1. HOW MUCH DO YOU REALLY WANT A BABY?

You want a baby. And the old tried and true, wham bam, pregnant ma'am, didn't work for you. You've even tried what you thought would be the magic bullet: in-vitro fertilization. And even that didn't work the first time.

I've been right where you are. No one wants to become an in-vitro Veteran. But here you are. I can tell you, you're in good company. Many a fine woman has stood right where you are. Unfortunately, there are lots of us out here. The up side is we're a pretty cool group. You will get through this, and you will be the stronger for it.

I offer my journey to you as a form of saying you're not alone. No matter how bad it gets, no matter how many emotionally induced roller coasters you must ride until you get to the end of your journey, be proud of who you are – even when you are at your worst.

I would also like to offer you a little hope because often there are happy endings – children at the end of the long dark IVF tunnel; your children. I connected with a group of about 20 women early on and out of that number, all but 2 are now moms. The other 2 women called an end to their search for children. Some adopted, some used donor eggs, donor sperm, both, neither, and any permutation you can think of. We all came to be Moms in our own unique way. And so will you.

I began my IVF journey when I was 44. I had my first child at age 46. What happened in between those points of time are contained in this book. This is not a story for the faint of heart. This is my journal – verbatim – raw - uncensored. The only things changed are, as they say, names, to protect the innocent. So prepare yourself for the blow by blow ordeal of one IVF veteran who lived to tell the tale.

So, if you're ready to begin accept the insanity because you are about to enter the ultimate intimate reality game:

In-vitro Fertilization.

2. IN THE BEGINNING

From my journal February, 2001.

Yesterday we got the news that one of the measurements of my husbands sperm, the morphology (shape), was a much lower percentage than normal. All along I was prepared for something to be screwy with my system. After all, I'm 44 and as a woman there's just so much more that can go wrong. So, I'd prepped myself emotionally, at least as much as you can, to get news that my eggs, or my something, weren't performing as they should. And in fact, that still may be the case. But now we know at least partly why, after several years of unprotected sex and more than a year of really trying for a baby, we have not met with success.

But sperm issues I was unprepared for. I was home alone when I called for the test results and the nurse who was looking at it for the first time, said, "Let's see, the Kruger is at 4 and we like to see 14 which means if you're going right to IVF you'll probably want to use ICSI and ... I stopped hearing for a moment. What was the Kruger? I couldn't remember. And what was ICSI? Again, no idea. Oh, I'd read the papers they'd sent home with us after our initial pre testing consultation. But all the high tech terms, well, they weren't going to apply to us anyway. I have a natural scientific curiosity about things as does my Chemist husband, but I just didn't want my mind to go there. We'd had those "what if" conversations but that was merely intellectual exercise with no emotions behind it. Some part of me tuned back into the phone conversation to ask, "How much would a round of In-Vitro Fertilization cost?" They'd have to have the money person call back. I had no real reaction yet, but immediately got online and went to my doctor's website to at least understand the terms. Kruger— the test to see how many normally shaped sperm there are. ICSI, Intracytoplasmic sperm injection. They could retrieve my eggs and inject some of the good sperm right into the egg…

Suddenly I was faced with the concept of going from simple mild assistance, you know, a little clomid to increase my egg production, maybe going so far as to wash and concentrate my husbands sperm and having it turkey basted into my uterus at the right time, to the ultimate high tech solution for reproduction.

I looked up IVF on the site, this time reading it as if it applied to me. The simple, we stimulate your ovaries to produce more than one egg, retrieve the eggs, fertilize them, and put them back into the uterus, sounded not so bad. The details were more daunting. 21 days of the pill, then on day 21 start 10-12 days of Lupron shots, then another approximately 9 days of intra muscular gonadotropin shots, the next day a hCG shot to stimulate ovulation. Two days later, egg pick up, an out patient procedure with anesthesia. Eggs are fertilized with ICSI. Some days later the embryos are transferred into the uterus. After all that I'm ordered to bed rest for 2 days which I'm absolutely sure I'd have no objections at that point. Progesterone is injected up until pregnancy is confirmed and if yes, then continued for a total of six weeks following embryo transfer and then for another 4 weeks by vaginal suppository. And then the possibility of more than one baby at a time....

My mind was reeling. I wondered if I really wanted to put myself through all that. Even while I was voicing my concerns deep inside I knew I would because the alternative was no children or adoption (problematic with our ages. I was already in my 40's and my husband is 20 years older than I). Then I came back to the original starting point, the sperm results. I had to tell my husband. Was he going to think himself less of a man? Since I'd already been prepared emotionally, knowing that part of me would fundamentally feel as if I'd failed as a woman if I could not produce offspring, I was pretty certain he'd have some reaction, even if he didn't show it outwardly.

I spent the afternoon trying to get in touch with how I felt so I could help my husband if he needed it. I found a reservoir of anger, not at my husband, but on a more basic level. Why, because of a male factor, did I, my body, have to go through all of these steps? No matter where the glitch in our mutual fertility occurred it was my body that would pay the price. Was this the penalty for being able to create within our bodies? I know this has always been so, and as my mom reminded me, men have in the past always been able to impregnate then walk away, while for women it was more than likely a life long effect. So, I saw myself as coming from this long line of women who carry this privilege/burden within their bodies. Here I was. Feeling a little sorry for myself.

The information seemed to affect my husband in two ways. Initially anger, which is his usual reaction to overwhelming emotional stimuli. And it ignited his fight or flight response—in this case the fight. He felt indignation that nothing was going to tell him he couldn't procreate. His desire for a child went up. He said if I was willing to go through IVF he felt there was a good chance he could vindicate himself. He wondered how this would affect his sex drive, would it go up as if he had something to really prove now?

I wondered if I now looked at him as less of a man, knowing I'm subjected to the same society of programming as anyone. Is male fertility equated to being a man? I know, as I sit here recording all this, that these are issues we're going to be dealing with as we embark on this journey.

Today I spoke with my mother. We tried to joke of multiple babies at once. Would she move in if we needed help? How would we handle twins or triplets?

I went for a long walk, trying to enjoy the first sun after a week of rain. In my mind I first thought about giving up my office space so mom, or whomever, could come and help out for 6 months. I resist that idea. My office/writing space is sacred to me. If I lost that would I go even more insane than just the normal insanity that comes with being first time parents? I know my husband feels the same way about his office. Perhaps if I redesigned the living room dining room area into a bedroom sitting room we could all have occasional privacy. Then there was the idea of putting the baby/babies into our master suite and leaving the guest room as a guest room. Was that wise? Healthy?

And then, there's the money issue. My husband teaches. Well, that means we're not rolling in the dough. And each round of IVF with ICSI and perhaps assisted egg hatching would cost up about $13,000—yikes! Where would that come from? How many rounds can we afford to go? If I have excess eggs the first time that can be frozen the price goes down considerably for the next procedure. Still…I tell myself, I know children are expensive. This is the least of it.

So on my walk today I come to the thought that, money issue aside, I'll mentally commit to 3 rounds, subject to change when we meet with the doctor in 10 days to go over all our options. I need a plan. Plans help me function. And my husband's a percentage player. He wants to know what are our odds each round? That will determine how far, how many…we kind of agree, if we can go a few rounds and have a better than 50/50 shot of success it's worth the emotional, physical, and financial investment.

I wonder, what if they inject the sperm but still no go? What if it's the sperm and egg both that don't work? Knowing my eggs are as mature as I, perhaps an anonymous donor egg and sperm from one of my brothers? Would that be too weird?

On and on the questions go in my mind. What if it doesn't work? What if it does and we have quintuplets? What about selective reduction? Could I, would I? If it was to help ensure the health of the remaining embryos, yes, probably. But if it was only because the thought of multiples is daunting, or as my friend says, a litter, is that reason enough? Would it be a risk to the other embryos?

And then my spiritual beliefs. If children are meant to be for us, wouldn't it just happen? Though if I broke a bone I wouldn't hesitate to use what science had to offer to mend it. Is this any different? Something is broken. Are we playing God/dess when we shouldn't? Or is all of this part of God/dess, meant for those of us who need a medical boost to achieve family?

I have no answers, even for myself at this point. And this is only the beginning.

March 6, 2001

Yesterday we met with the doctor. Reality check. As it turns out it really doesn't matter about my husband's sperm—all we need are a few good ones and even with his percentage there are still thousands to choose from. I admit that my anger at the male female thing has reared up big time. According to statistics, the success of in-vitro is related to the age of my eggs, in fact it's a rather dauntingly low percentage. He told us 8-25% and of course I get stuck on the 8% and I know this doctor's stats are higher than many. The book we have says IVF with ICSI for women over 40 is 5-10%. That's lots of money and emotional investment with not a great chance. Donor eggs is an answer. Young, nonwrinkled, unscarred, vigorous eggs. I can't tell you how much that thought depresses me. I want my own DNA passed on. I know, many mothers will tell you that it doesn't matter. Motherhood is motherhood. But I, and my husband, seem to have considerably less enthusiasm when we consider being parents without my genetics involved. We can only afford 2 rounds of IVF. In 3 days the doctor will do a mock transfer—a practice session for placing the eggs in my uterus. Then next week, when my cycle begins I'll start on birth control pills and then on fertility drugs for super ovulation. How my ovaries respond to those drugs will determine if we go a complete cycle or not.

I don't know why. Usually I'm one of those that look at odds and decides they don't apply to me. And I'm usually right. In this case I find myself believing them—that my chances are slim. I'm depressed and have this heavy sense of grief, as if it's already failed. Does this mean it will? Should I not do it? I don't know why I'm depressed. It hasn't not worked yet!

3. INTERMISSION
IVF SUPERSTITIONS

Things rumored to increase your chances for successful IVF
— all of which, at one time or another, have been tried by
desperate IVF veterans.

FOOD/DRINK

- Eat pineapples
- Eat Papaya
- Eat Nuts
- Don't eat nuts
- Drink green tea
- Drink black tea
- Don't drink tea
- Eat yams
- Sip wine
- Get drunk
- Don't Drink

SUPERSTITIONS

- Never ever let your cat sleep on your lap as it might make your uterus too warm
- If you want 2 children plant 2 rose bushes and say hello to them every morning
- Get drunk
- Don't move a muscle for 3 days after your transfer
- Pretend you never had a transfer
- Sing lullabies to your up-until-now empty womb
- Get a massage
- Pray
- Curse God
- Cry like a baby
- Buy maternity clothes
- Buy baby clothes
- Get rid of baby clothes and anything having to do with babies
- Paint the nursery
- Hang booties over the entrance to intended nursery
- Nail the nursery shut
- Have sex
- Don't let a penis near you
- Fall in love with your fertility doctor
- Hate your fertility doctor
- Name your new dog after your fertility doctor
- Have an orgasm the night before a transfer
- Get really really sick the day of transfer
- Plan a big expensive trip with nonrefundable tickets
- Assume the worst
- Assume the best
- I saved this one for last as it might actually really work: Acupuncture before and during your IVF cycle.

4. MY REAL EMOTIONAL JOURNEY BEGINS

Cycles 1&2
Day 1 March 16, 2001

I'm so anxious. Two days ago I had some spotting so I immediately called the docs office to say it was day one and I needed to come in on day 3 (today). Spotting stopped. My period didn't start until today. I feel disappointed with myself that it didn't start when I wanted it to. What does it matter? Except that I'm anxious to get going…plus I took the birth control pill this morning—I thought I'd gotten instructions to start it on day 1. Turns out I was supposed to wait until I saw the nurse practitioner. I feel like I did something wrong. I need to relax a little in all this or I'm going to drive myself crazy. We'll probably give them the money for 1 cycle today. And they're supposed to go over the entire approximately 40 day cycle so we know exactly what to expect when. Too Late. I'm already crazy. Surrender to the universe. That's my mantra for the day.

Postponed. Favorite Baby Names.

April 9, 2001

We had to postpone everything. When we went in last month we were told that my Rubella vaccination had worn off—in other words I have no immunity to Rubella. Not a problem except if I'm exposed to it when I'm pregnant. I wrestled with myself. Do I do the vaccination and wait for 3 months? I was so geared up and ready to go. If I'm honest, frantic is the right word. My husband, being the voice of reason, said this is something we can control. So I went ahead and had the vaccination which means embryo transfer cannot occur for 90 days after that—which is June 21. Now, since it's a 40+ day cycle this means that we can probably start with the pill on my May cycle.

Since we postponed I feel terrible. It's as if I wanted to barrel ahead so I couldn't give things much thought and now I'm forced to watch the calendar days go slowly by. On top of that we have to make sure we don't get pregnant so now after all this time of gearing up for my fertile time we now have to avoid it—or take certain precautions. I'm going through my days, writing some, marketing, generally giving the appearance of living my life. But inside there is really only one thing. baby. baby baby baby. When? My internal tuning fork is already set to June and I find myself doing what I despise in others—biding my time. Not really living fully. I tell myself to be in the here and now but they are only words and my heart is beating for motherhood. Outwardly I'm still my relatively calm self, though more moody than usual. Who would know inside I'm a cesspool of conflicting emotions? My husband and I pass some of the time joking about names. I really like Quasar. He says he doesn't want to do that to a kid. We joke about what if it's quintuplets? Do we name them all after one category? Spices? Rosemary, Sage, Cinnamon, Nutmeg, and Marjoram. Or famous people? William Tecumseh (family name) and Betsy Ross. Flowers? Rose, Tulip…you get the idea. I'm a science fiction writer. I like Quasar, Nova, Pulsar, Star and Borealis. Or ancient Gods and Goddesses…Thor and Aphrodite and Isis…my husband is more practical. Jack, Bill, Jeff, Mary, and Marie. These are the moments when we smile and laugh. And how will we fit 5 cribs in the room? These conversations are fun and funny for us. Much needed during this challenging time.

So for now, I labor only at everyday living, not giving birth. My friend says I'm suffering from prepartum depression. I'm depressed a lot. Tired. Weary. Full of longing. It's getting so I can't even stand myself. I know I'm poor company. And even though my husband is willing to talk it's my body, my cycles, my hormones that sweep me away. He can't ever know what it's like to carry this inside a female body. I don't want to become one of those women who only thinks and talks about baby this and baby that. But inside, the simple truth is, I am. I may control it on the outside but inside it's all there is. I'm obsessed with the health channel on television, baby stories, medical stories about babies, fertility profiles…any and everything having to do with babies and giving birth. I cry. I sleep. And I wait. I can't believe this is me.

We Try to Cycle. The Drugs.

May 17, 2001

At last we've begun. Really begun. I started taking the pill yesterday on day 3 of my cycle. On June 1, I start Lupron injections and then it spirals up from there. More drugs and shots than I originally knew. I already know I'll feel like a pin cushion. My best friend is excited about the kid thing now. We keep talking about triplets and I imagine how that would be—the challenge, the difficulty, the joy of those varied personalities all developing.

As it turns out this agonizing pause of some weeks has been good for my soul. There is a calm in my center where before was the desperate yearning for babies now now now. I am anxious of course but I'm enjoying this phase. It's as if someone came to me and said you'll be pregnant in some weeks. Prepare. So that's what I've been doing. All those things in the house I never did after we moved that were on my list. I painted the master bathroom (it looks fabulous I must say—like an Italian Fresco—warm and alive yet easy to look at). We got some new hand me down furniture. Cleaned the garage. And of course have contingency plans for one, two, and three babies. I've spoken to my mom about her helping. I have a list of women who will be here to assist particularly if I have multiples. I've even researched what happens when you have multiples—the potential for long term bed rest. With that in mind I'm doing things now BECAUSE I CAN. I think this helps keep me hopeful. I don't hesitate to jump in and do and enjoy the very act of doing. This is how we should all live life, full enjoyment of each phase for the next one will be different. This one is so big, from no kids to kids, that you can't miss it but shouldn't each phase, day, of life be perceived as such? For the truth is everything ends. Each thing will come and go and we should enjoy it for what it is. Right now, my last days without pregnancy, without children. It's a time of wonder and a time I am now at ease with, inside myself.

Today we went for another scan to check my ovaries—toknow what's there before we begin. This is the first of many scans. And the schedule. So complex. Drugs for 5 days, 9 days, 17 days, over-lapping days, that I made a calendar on my computer—put a stork next to June and clip art baby pictures—one screaming, one sleeping, one sitting quietly with a stuffed bear—that covers the possibilities. Doesn't it? And it's an attempt to make it fun, to make myself smile when I look on the fridge to see how many times I'll be poked by needles that day. For July, I put pregnancy at the top and a couple possible dates for pregnancy confirmation. Though the egg retrieval and embryo transfer are scheduled for June 22 and June 25 or 27 respectively, I didn't want the calendar to stop in June. Superstitious I guess. Making the statement that it goes on after the embryo transfer. In fact, that's only the beginning. And perhaps we'll keep a calendar throughout the entire pregnancy, sort of quick glance journal.

Starting the cycle makes me feel more proactive. However for now, I'll enjoy our childless state as I know it's coming to an end. Now there is time. Time for long hot baths, time for walks, time for self.

<u>Anger and Depression.</u>

June 7, 2001

There's a black cloud in my head filling me with anger and depression. This is the 7th day of Lupron 10u and the last day of the pill. I was actually feeling okay up until 3 days ago when the bad mood suddenly hit. This feels so unlike me and I've completely lost perspective on the connection between these shots and babies. Though the shots themselves are not particularly painful there is something about having your soft underbelly violated that's psychologically difficult. Its soft delicate skin is meant for caressing not puncturing.

The day we started the Lupron, the doctor found a rather large cyst so now I have to go back in tomorrow to see if I'm going to have to have it aspirated on Monday. That depressed me. On the up side, the mock transfer went much smoother this time.

It's my anger that bothers me most. Everything is irritating and it's all I can do not to tear my husband a new you know what. He's kind, giving me the shots, but everything he does feels wrong right now. For that matter, I feel that way about everyone right now. This is definitely foreign to how I normally feel. Is my anger coming from fear of failure? Fear of success? Both? I feel as if I'm mourning the old me, the me I've always been. And even though I so much want these children, that little girl in me who doesn't want the responsibility, the little girl who didn't even like dolls, is throwing tantrums. I'm trying to let her feel how she feels even as it fills me with a mass of conflicting emotions. I wonder how other women feel when they go through these phases. I feel cut off, alone. I have supportive friends who listen and help but it's still my body going through all this. I feel this IVF is going to be successful and in that sense this is only the beginning. Maybe that's why it's so hard. Things will never be the same. And I want that. Yet I don't. Is this how it feels to be a wishy washy woman? Kids are the one thing you can never walk away from and I've often walked away from careers, men, homes. It's part of why I must do this. And part of why it's so hard.

Today I saw the cutest 6 month old at the post office. He was smiling and charming everyone. It's amazing how they can captivate an entire room. The mother was young, slim, and healthy. I envied her youth and found myself automatically assuming she had no problem getting pregnant. I waited years so there are more blips in the road.

I watched a squirrel this morning eating a green nectarine from our tree.

I hate feeling this way. I hate myself right now. And the world.

Argh, Hormone Hell.

June 11, 2001

I've become hormonally challenged. This morning my husband woke me at 5 so we could begin the next phase— stimulation drugs. No as fun as it sounds. What it means is now 5 shots a day, as we've added heparin 2x per day to thin blood and help prevent clots and Follistin and Pergonal which is an intramuscular shot (in the butt). Lupron continues at half the previous dose.

The news on Friday was good. The cyst was gone and my blood tests came back with an estradiol level of 18 which gave us the go ahead to begin this morning. So, the news is all good but I feel so not like myself. I can feel an immediate change with the shots this morning. Now my head feels hot inside as if there is pressure and my energy feels, well, rounder. It does seem as if this is a more proactive phase. The stuff before was to shut my system down, a rest before the sprint if you will. Now we're beginning the sprint. I had a weird thought that perhaps humans are striving for the time when they can tell their ovaries to ripen/produce the desired number of eggs instead of just one. Maybe IVF is a way to show the body how to reprogram itself. Reaching for science fiction to make myself feel better, perhaps?

My next appt. is Fri. A blood test, again for estradiol, and then a scan to see how I'm responding to the stimulation.

Last Friday I met with the IVF coordinator. She was full of tidbits and after I told her my husband and I wanted to bring the sperm in with us the morning of egg retrieval she shared some funny stories with me—as in don't put the specimen on the heater or air conditioning in the car. We talked more about the things that I can't do. Starting now. No more wine. Sigh. No caffeine, not a problem, I drink decaf. No chocolate. Also not a problem for me. No baths. I'm not sure if that starts now or after the embryo transfer. That's a real tough one for me. I live for my baths. Even belonged to a bath of the month club. No lifting anything over 10 lbs. Also tough as I'm always doing the heavy house stuff. No intercourse. Until after the first trimester. Yikes! The thing they tell me to avoid here is penetration. Back to being a teen and "the everything but" routine…

It seems a little harder to breathe today. Due to shot? The stress of thinking about the shot? I'm definitely stressed. A skin rash on my arm, a zit on my butt. My body's talking and it's none too thrilled about some of this. At least I have a supportive system. My dreams are wild, nightmarish things. This morning I was crying when I woke.

This is a wild ride, one I wasn't prepared for. The intellectualthoughts have no relationship to the real deal. I'm glad I work for myself and don't have to go 'out in public right now. My mind feels as if it's under water. 11 days to egg retrieval. But who's counting?

June 13, 2001

I've recruited family and friends to do a meditation/prayer on June 21st at 6pm for 10 minutes-geared toward, of course, successful outcome - meaning healthy pregnancy leading to healthy baby/s. This is the first time my family has ever done anything like this so that's pretty cool.

I'm trying to bring myself around to a better attitude and stop feeling like my body is being assaulted. An image from the Gandhi movie popped into my mind—the moment when the men are being clubbed and it "goes on and on into the night." That's what my body feels like. I know that's silly in the sense that this is a good thing. I want this, or at least the end result of this. We don't create any experience we're not in agreement to so on certain levels this is the way I want to get pregnant. Hmm. My husband is trying his best but when it hurts he gets the blame.

My head is clouded and I know I'm not thinking clearly. I went out to run a few errands today and wondered if I was sharp enough to be driving. Slow reactions, my mind wanders and it's hard to make decisions.

I thought I would be joyful doing this, knowing what I'm doing it for. How much of this emotional response is due to the hormones being injected? I know no one likes to be injected; still, it's not as if I have a terminal disease or something. THIS IS A GOOD THING!

June 14, 2001

A quote I saw yesterday, "Only parts suffer, not the whole."

I am doing much better. Amazing what deciding to have a better attitude can do. With each shot now I think, "one shot closer to being pregnant." I am starting to feel my ovaries, kind of a full, pressurized feeling. Tomorrow we go in for the scan. We means, my friend C is driving me down. She's my back up husband. Maybe the shift in hormones is making me feel better too. I actually did some gardening this morning—nothing heavy, just trimming. I do get tired more easily but it felt good to be out there.

Stymied Again.

June 17, 2001

On my June 15 appointment I got really cruddy news.
Couldn't even write about it until now. My ovaries weren't
responding to the stimulation drugs so we had to pull the
plug on the cycle. I feel such loss, pain anger. Yesterday I
spent most of the day crying. I know this doesn't spell the
end but I feel ended. Whenever I start my next cycle we'll try
again with a different protocol—no suppression. I'm afraid
to try again. Afraid of going through this again. So much
body assault to lead to nothing. My stomach is still really
bruised. I look like I went many rounds with Muhammed Ali
in his prime. I know somewhere in here there must be some
good but right now I'm pissed at the universe for all the
heads up signs and now this. Thank the Goddess that my
friend C was there when we got the news. She was stunned. I
went numb right away, as if a large wave of "this can't be"
was battling reality and it was too much. As she drove us
home we held hands and cried. Crap. I'd much rather have
been Thelma and Louise going off the cliff at that moment.
There is still part of me that doesn't believe the news, and I
find myself actually missing getting the shots because with
the shots there is hope. Now hope for this cycle is ended and
I feel tragedy.

Today I feel as if I got hit by a Mack truck and though I
went for a long walk this morning my energy is about nil. I'm
confused and angry and hurt and feel such loss, as if the
undeveloped eggs died. Is the loss of potential any different
than the loss of the actual? If I had to have loss this no

doubt is better than having gone to the end and then having it not work.

For now, I'll let myself grieve and when I'm ready I'll look to trying again. This is a wild, difficult, ride.

5. INTERMISSION
A TRUE SEPT.11 STORY

Picture it: Era – post 9/11. Everyone was scared. Security heightened, worry flowed like so much sewage, choking the joy out of simple pleasures.

Enter IVF veteran we'll call Infertile Myrtle. She innocently boards a plane bound for…well, the location does not matter. Like all the other passengers that day she roughly shoved her bag into the overhead compartment, pushing it way back so it would not inadvertently shift and be poised ready to smash her head upon arrival.

But her purse with its secret precious cargo was another matter entirely. This she tucked gently between her feet on the floor then touched it tenderly – as if she were touching a baby on the forehead. She glanced at her watch and paid no attention to preflight safety information.

She leaned back in her seat, adjusted the belt, and then shut her eyes. Some minutes later the pilot announced they would be delayed about twenty minutes. Her eyes flew open and she swore. She made herself look out the window but her eyes kept coming back to her watch.

Her nervous actions caught the attention of the passenger across the aisle, a well-dressed gentleman who watched her from the corner of his eye.

Finally the plane pulled out and headed down the runway. Airborne at last. As soon as the captain turned off the seatbelt sign she picked up her purse, popped off the belt and moved quickly down the narrow isle. She got to the bathroom only to find it occupied. "Damn it to hell." She looked at her watch, watched the bathroom for a moment, then moved secretively to the empty space next to the closet. She huddled over her purse, and looked around to make sure no one was watching. She flipped open her bag and pulled out a sharp object.

"Watch out!" a woman screamed. That lady has a knife!"

Infertile Myrtle looked up, her eyes searching desperately for the lady with the knife. She saw no one. In the next moment she was shoved violently against the wall of the plane and the well dressed gentleman from across the aisle` slammed her arm behind her.

"Drop it!" He forced her hand open. The needle slipped from her fingers.

"Wait – I have to use that!" She tried to pull free, her eyes on the needle.

The man stepped on it. "I'll bet."

"You don't understand – it's my progesterone! I need it now! I'm in cycle!" Poor Infertile Myrtle, simply trying to shoot up on schedule.

A flight attendant searched her purse and found a copy of the prescription. After much explaining to a bunch of fertile folk, they set her free. She didn't care about almost landing in jail. All she hoped was that injecting late wouldn't mess up her IVF schedule.

6. LOST HOPE

June 21, 2001

I'm spending a lot of time alone, quiet time. Long exhausting walks and lots of gardening. I'm still really sad—far more than this situation warrants. Could be partly hormonal I suppose. I seem to be getting mild hot flashes as my body settles back to normal. I feel as if I'm going through a rearrangement of self. I'm craving quiet time and am reading again. I stopped for some weeks—just not in the mood which is weird for me. There is something inside, as if I'm searching for my own power within as I pull away from outside sources. This is a good thing. I think with such good sources of information at my disposal I've started going external too quickly and losing part of that me that is so strong and can create and figure things for myself. This is the beauty of 'tragedy' in that it makes you look at yourself even amidst the grief. The fact that I am sadder than I would have thought tells me there is more going on beneath that I am not conscious of.

I've temporarily stopped watching the baby shows on the health channel. I don't think seeing babies makes me sad but I do need a break from such intense focus. I'm a bit adrift as so much of my attention and energy was directed toward making a baby. I didn't plan for this delay (duh), so now I have no commitments, have pulled back from writing as much. But I'm still keeping myself in low gear since it's so hard for me to get here I'll take advantage in trying to give myself some true downtime instead of just pretend downtime. My brain is even quieter these days and that's a special break. I haven't cried in two days so I know I'm healing from this sudden surprise.

<u>Back on the Baby Train.</u>

July 24, 2001

Back on the baby train. I went down to doc yesterday and got the new schedule. Injections start the 31st with proposed egg retrieval on the 13th. I'm glad we're moving into it fast but I have such a mixed bag of emotions going into this one. Fear, that it won't work again and I'll have to once more feel as if my body fails me. I want this so much. Today, an email from my brother that his girlfriend is pregnant. Their first just turned one year. According to him they had one day of unprotected sex. He tried for years to have a child in previous relationships, and went through the whole IVF thing without success. So it's not like his road to children was easy, still, this news evokes in me a terrible angry streak of jealousy and the sensation of "Not fair!" I want to be happy for him/them if this is what they want. But I have so much to offer, don't I too deserve to experience my own children? How many other women have cried over this same thought, feeling…my life is blessed. I have so much but why does this basic fundamental aspect, the most basic thing to existence there is, elude me? Us? Please, let this time work. Let us have our own children without having to wait more. I know things happen, or don't happen, and we don't always know the whys but as I read somewhere, if this is not meant to be, then please Goddess, take my desire away so I don't have to suffer so. I want to be pregnant; I want to experience giving birth, breastfeeding, smelling my/our baby's head, teaching and learning, family, the pain and joy, the hard work, the play. It's hard to write this through the blur of my tears which are running hot down my cheeks.

July 31, 2001

My husband got home last night from a two week trip and we happily headed down to San Diego to see the doc as we were scheduled to begin the next cycle. We brought the Lupron with us as instructed.. Dr. B stuck the transducer up my who-who, a procedure that has become all too routine for me at this point—I've never been terribly modest but with this I've forgotten that I'm exposing a private part—it's so much the least of it all. Anyway, he sees that there are two developing eggs. Isn't this great! I think. I can produce more than one egg…however, one is already at 12, I assume these are millimeters, as he measures it on the screen, and the other at 8. Well, the one at 12 is too big for me to start Lupron because it will more than likely develop into a Lupron cyst. He says, we may have to wait another cycle. I'm thinking, No! I realize he's going away in Sept. so this might be a two cycle wait…no, no, and again no. The pill was supposed to suppress any egg development…how is this possible? What he decides is that we should come back tomorrow, on the 1st, to recheck. If it's no bigger we'll consider moving forward…maybe. As so as he leaves the examine room, I swear. As My husband and I drive home I go on and on about how everything in me is screaming not to wait. I wonder, out loud, if we could harvest these two eggs. Aren't two better than none? Even if that is little bang for our buck…or maybe wait another week and start? Can the schedule be messed with that much?

I spend the afternoon and evening, stressing, going through mental hell. Why am I doing this to myself? I talk to my body and to my ovaries. I attempt to absorb the too large egg, or to ovulate it. Anything, so we can try.

Aug. 1, 2001

With much trepidation we return to the docs in the afternoon. He, once more sticks the transducer up my who-who, and the picture is much different today. The egg seems to have already formed into a cyst, and most importantly, split from my ovary. That's good news. An ovarian Lupron cyst mucks up a cycle but if it's not on the ovary, not a problem. So, he also sees a couple eggs that measure 5…this is good, at least for me. They like to see 4 on each side but considering my no egg cycle last time I'm pleased, even if he's not. In any case, we get the go ahead. And we're still on the same schedule, it's just that we have 1.5 days less of the Lupron injections. This cycle protocol is different. It's called a microflare. There's no suppression first so it's much quicker. And it's only Lupron, in a very small dose which promotes stimulation not suppression, and Follistim, no pergonal. If all goes well the egg retrieval will be on Aug. 13.

Aug. 5, 2001

Four days into Follistim injections. This time we're doing them subcue so all the shots are in my stomach. We've started the Heparin, too. So it's six shots a day in the belly. To top it off I got attacked by a flesh-eating ant the other night, on my stomach, so between the red welts from the bites and the injection site bruises my stomach looks like a war zone. Though the Follistim needle doesn't hurt near as much when it's subcue, the burning of the Follistim when it goes in can be nearly unbearable. It spreads out in these arcs of burning sharp pain that can last for up to an hour. At least for me. Last night my husband was reading the information that comes with Follistim and it said that if you massage the area after the injection it can cut down on the discomfort and help the absorption. So, we tried that this morning. Hurt like a....but the discomfort did go away faster.

Today I'm pretending to do some normal things, fixed the BBQ, worked on a jigsaw puzzle, and watched the hummingbirds. But my thoughts are mostly on one thing— the appointment tomorrow when we see if this time, please Goddess, I have eggs. I do feel more discomfort this time, though it's hard to say for the red hot burning itch of the ant bites are making me kind of sick. I always react to insect bites with a sort of allergic response and my pale skin gets so red. Anyway, I'm doing a fair amount of lying around and watching bad television.

Aug. 6, 2001

Finally! Some good news. I was so stressed going to the doctors today I felt nauseated. However, there are eggs! And he was particularly excited about my uterine lining—he said I have a B pattern. "Give me a lining of this pattern and one good embryo and I can get a woman pregnant every time." Not that I'll be hanging onto those words much….

I'm so relieved I feel ill. I don't know how else to explain it. Should I print up a large banner and hang it in the wind for all to see? Eggs, eggs, beautiful eggs.

Now we go back Thursday to see the eggs again and determine which day the egg retrieval will be. It's scheduled for Monday at this point. My body is tired and achy and my abdomen area is full of pressure/discomfort but since we got home I've had this hyper energy which I've been feeding off of..

Hold this miracle space.

Aug. 16, 2001

Damn it. Gone and gone. My left ovary just isn't showing the activity and on the right side one is already most likely too large. Doc said if we want to try at all we have to trigger with HCG tonight and attempt recovery Saturday though he says our chances of getting any viable eggs is 1 in a 1000. I'm ignoring the odds.

Took HCG trigger shot at 11 p.m.

Aug. 17, 2001

Am spending most of this day crying. Having hope dangled in our face and then taken away again seems crueler than no hope at all.

Aug. 18, 2001

Spent the night at a hotel last night to be closer to the hospital because we wanted to bring the sperm in with us. This whole thing feels so clinical I wanted at least a small connection to the sperm.

I was put under at 10am and the next thing I remember was hearing a couple of nurses talking—"How many eggs did they get?" "None." "Wow. That doesn't happen very often."

I knew they were talking about me and it was confirmed of course when my husband came in—I could tell by his sigh before he even spoke. I tried to wake up but felt really creepy coming out of the anesthetic and that was probably due in part to knowing it had all been for nothing. Doc has aspirated 3 follicles, 2 from right, one from left, but gotten nothing but cellular debris.

Spent the ride home in the car trying to think about anything but the reality of it all because if I let myself cry I was afraid I wouldn't be able to stop.

Aug. 19, 2001

Woke up feeling like crap. My father, a retired anesthesiologist and his wife, came down to visit though they had no idea we'd done the egg retrieval yesterday. I felt so lousy I couldn't make myself get out of bed so let my husband deal with them when they first arrived. It dawned on me as I was lying there that I was waiting until my husband told them what had happened because if I had to speak the story I would have a breakdown. After I finally did come downstairs I felt better because conversation was a good distraction.

My older brother called in the evening—he was so sympathetic I thought I might implode with unshed grief.

7. INTERMISSION: A POEM
DAMN IT, I WANT A BABY

How I want a baby,

I want one oh so bad,

That every time I see a mom

I get so very mad.

I've tried and tried to get knocked up

The good old fashioned way,

But nothing ever did the trick

Now it's come what may.

The doctor prods and pokes at me

And tests for god knows what,

Then gives me packs of drugs and things

To shoot right in my butt.

He wields a sinful cooter cam

And other fancy gear,

I try and smile and make small talk

While my gut is full of fear.

This has to work it costs so much

I wonder how we'll pay,

All I think is baby this, baby that,

every single day.

I thought in vitro'd work right away

I feel so desperate now,

I'd give it up if I thought I could

But I really don't know how.

I want "me" back, but where am I?

Buried oh so deep,

I'd tell you what I really think

But there'd have to be a bleep.

8. DONOR EGGS?

Aug. 25, 2001

This week has gone by in a haze of depression, anger, and fatigue, though decisions have been made. I kept wondering why the universe would tease me with what looked like a possible cycle with my eggs and then take it away. I would have been better off emotionally if I hadn't responded at all on the 2nd cycle, as in the first.

After Monday I at least felt like I could talk about it. I spoke with my younger brother and we talked abstractly about donor eggs. I was still in a bad way and it was a hard conversation for me. By Tuesday I was thinking we'd try one more cycle on me and if that didn't work we'd go to donor eggs. I was really focused on wanting my own genetics and being angry with my husband that he didn't have to face this. Even with the male factor his sperm can still be injected into the eggs.

I thought of the money and how we're draining our entire savings for this. If I do one more cycle with my eggs then we'll be below zero in our accounts if we then had to do a donor cycle.

I thought of adoption, thinking that at least then my husband wouldn't be able to lay more claim than me on the child and we'd also be guaranteed a child after spending the money. Then I thought of using donor eggs and my brother's sperm. That idea I liked and would have far less hesitation. My husband of course would then have to deal with not being genetically connected. Then, I thought, let's do donor eggs, and inject half with my husband's sperm and half with one of my brother's put them in and let nature take its course. I felt myself getting more and more angry as the hours passed until we sat and talked through all the ins and outs. My body is grieving and it's VERY hard to let go of the concept of that link—the drive to pass on our genes is about the strongest drive there is. My husband and I talked about nature vs. nurture. We both could say that the top priority in all this was to have the experience of raising a child.

I spoke long hours to my friends—my closest friend told me point blank she thought my ego was getting in the way of my thinking - wasn't the important thing the spirit of the child, not the cells? I know she's right....

My 2nd cousin, whom I'm very close to (she taught me to tie my shoes when I was little) has two adopted children. I talked and talked with her about her coming to that decision so many years ago. Of course, back then donor eggs were not a possibility. That reminded me to be grateful this option exists instead of angry I have to consider this.

And finally, I got on the internet and found a message board with women who'd gone through this very thing. I found I was certainly not alone. Every emotion, every thought, was normal. Including the anger and jealousy toward my husband. I even have thoughts of jealousy that my husband's sperm are going to fertilize another woman's eggs. I mentioned that to my sister-in-law and she said to remember they would be at that point, my eggs, I'd paid for them. I said it's true, when I buy a shirt I consider it mine, not the store it came from. Perhaps a crass way of looking at it but somehow that made it easier.

Today I called the fertility clinic and said I decided to go straight to donor eggs. Bang for the buck, that's the best shot we have if I'd like to be pregnant and experience pregnancy and motherhood. I talked a long time to the receptionist and she had many things to say that were very helpful. Next Friday we go in to do a preliminary look a donor pictures and then we'll get details on those we are interested in. Then we'll meet with the doctor.

I feel split. It's as if my spirit is making the decisions and we're moving ahead. But my body is still so very sad and tears are only a breath away. I think this grieving will take a long time but I think once I'm pregnant it'll go away because I'll be seeing things in a new way, as a mother, and it won't matter where the genes came from. In reading comments from other women who have been through this I know this will happen. As one friend said to me (she had kids long ago) "Once you carry something inside you and give birth to it, even if it's a shoe you'd love it."

So, I continue to ponder nature vs. nurture, and work on getting the anger from my space and in the meantime my husband and I are going to visit my one year old niece to get some baby fun in. This is really hard and I often feel it's a bad dream. In that moment just after waking, before full consciousness, I almost forget all the bad stuff. But then it comes and admittedly, these days, getting up is hard. I don't pop out of bed to greet the day but tend to stare a lot and wonder what to do with myself.

I think sometimes I'm a very selfish person and wonder if part of this journey, for me, is to confront the basic essence of unconditional love in a way that challenges me. I don't have any answers, just thoughts and tears, and yes, a bit of excitement that there's still a good chance I will experience motherhood.

9. PICKING A DONOR

Sept. 3, 2001

Well, the stress of picking a donor—in bad moments I think of it as a replacement for myself—made me sick. Just starting to get better from a bad chest cold—literally lost my voice for a couple days which I took to mean I was supposed to stop talking and listen for awhile.

My husband and I went through pictures together after looking at some basic facts, age, height, weight, hair and eye color, body build, skin tone, education. He is really looking for fair skin like mine. Not too many red heads to pick from…anyway we came away with a few possibles and over the course of many days I continued to look and think. I had a few badly photocopied photos to look at. My close friend came by to give her opinion and we were able to pretty easily narrow it down to three possible donors. There were a few others I wanted to see…finally on the 30th I went back to make a final decision even though I could barely talk. But I figured I would start feeling better once the choice was made. By then my first choice was obvious and I also have my second choice. Now we're waiting to hear if my top pick is available and ready.

This is a weird difficult time. I'm anxious to move forward but I'm still so sad I won't be able to have my genetics involved. That's a drive so basic to our essence I suppose it can't ever be truly gone. And I know these will be my children it's just that at this point all I have is the going in stress without the good feelings of being pregnant and having my child/ren inside of me so I can start to know them/their spirit.

I spend a lot of time lying around not knowing how I feel. Should I be pursuing having kids so hard? Do all these obstacles mean that we aren't supposed to have children? Or is this the journey…it's so hard to tell in life whether obstacles are put in your path because you're on the wrong path or whether they are there because they are something you are meant to overcome, defining part of who you become? Is letting go of the genetic connection part of learning unselfish love for me? Sometimes I feel as if I know a lot about myself and the world spiritually. And other times I don't seem to know a thing and can only go through each day stumbling blindly forward and trusting that in the end it will work as it's supposed to and that the not knowing is part of the process.

In all of this it's so easy to lose the we of this. The entire IVF process is straining, to say the very least, on a relationship. We've weathered okay though intimacy is rare and hard to come by. There's always something in the middle, be it injected hormones, or emotional stress, or fear.

I think now, of this potential egg lady—gene lady. Who is she to me? Our Karma? Is the only way I can bring the children I truly want to me to use her eggs? If my eggs worked would it not be as I really want? This gene lady is in ways I can only know on paper, much like me, in her hobbies, her intelligence. And yes, her red hair. Even better in some ways. Taller. Is this a convoluted way of improving myself and what I can offer my children?

So, we wait, I wonder. And we wait.

Sept. 5, 2001

Yesterday I talked with the nurse and found out that they couldn't reach my top donor pick. But number two is excited and ready to start. I don't know as much about her, though I do know she is blond and doesn't have red hair. And though I told myself that if first choice was supposed to work it would, and if not to be content with my second pick. Still, this sent me into another emotional spin. No red hair? Not even that? (at least blond hair, blue eyes) Could I in all of this not have even one thing I'd like? Even though I know donor hair color doesn't necessarily mean the kid/s will have that color as they may have my husband's. Still…it's as if this is making it real and I'm afraid again. Do I really want to do this? I know I do but… when I start to think about things like this I try and think about how I'll feel if this doesn't work—how at that point I would think back and realize how unimportant hair color is. At least now there is all this hope, how well donor cycles work, how high the chances are…and if we should ever have to move into considering adoption how I'll miss thinking of this chance to carry our child/ren.

Sometimes thinking that puts this in perspective. Still, the body urge does not go away so I try and compartmentalize that. Allow the feeling but separate it from the wanting of children.

We have this last month for a miracle—a "natural" fertilization and implantation…with my own genes…I don't really have any hope of this but still it's there, lurking…one more try….

I've been spending lots of time reading the bulletin boards at one of the IVF sites—particularly the section with donor eggs. All these women going through the same thing. It's so hard, and it's so miraculous.

I still have the faint markings of bruises on my stomach from the last cycle. We got the bill…yikes. My body is in a low state of energy, more than the recent cold, as this year has been very difficult for it. I wonder when I look back how I'll feel about this year.

Yesterday I did have a glimpse of something. If we're programmed genetically to be a certain way, which is reinforced as the baby develops, what happens when the genes don't match the mother's? Interesting philosophical question. Will they be more free and unrestricted by the structure of heritage so that they're better able to follow their own path? Now that would be something…and perhaps the reason, beyond biology, that father's can now have children (even with poor sperm) because of ICSI, is that they don't carry the children so it's let's critical that they release the genetic link? Spiritual food for thought.

Sept. 11, 2001

Disaster today. Terrorists hijacked planes and flew them into targets—the world trade center, the pentagon, and the last crashed in PA. I'm stunned and very sad. There are so many things far worse than infertility.

Weirdly, life is going on despite the terrible events in New York. I started my period today and called the clinic. My donor had also started and has done her FSH testing though we don't know results yet. I'm to call in a couple days to find out and I may start the pill this cycle though the donor is not going to—which means we're not really starting this cycle, but next. Best as I can figure that puts my embie transfer at end of November, beginning of December. I was hoping to start sooner of course but trying to take it as it comes. I don't do that very well with this stuff...I wonder what the donor is thinking and feeling right now.

Been spending a bit of each day on the IVF site and it's so great to connect with a group of women who are going through this also. You can talk with family and friends but no one gets what it's really like.

10. INTERMISSION: PRAYER AND IVF

Question:

Does prayer influence the success of in vitro fertilization-embryo transfer?

There was a study done in 2001 —

OBJECTIVE: To assess the potential effect of intercessory prayer (IP) on pregnancy rates in women being treated with in vitro fertilization-embryo transfer (IVF-ET). STUDY DESIGN: Prospective, double-blind, randomized clinical trial in which patients and providers were not informed about the intervention. Statisticians and investigators were masked until all the data had been collected and clinical outcomes were known. The setting was an IVF-ET program at Cha Hospital, Seoul, Korea. IP was carried out by prayer groups in the United States, Canada and Australia. The investigators were at a tertiary medical center in the United States. The patients were 219 women aged 26-46 years who were consecutively treated with IVF-ET over a four-month period. Randomization was performed after stratification of variables in two groups: distant IP vs. no IP. The clinical pregnancy rates in the two groups were the main outcome measure.

RESULTS: After clinical pregnancies were known, the data were unmasked to assess the effects of IP after assessment of multiple comparisons in a log-linear model. The IP group had a higher pregnancy rate as compared to the no-IP rate (50% vs. 26%, $P = .0013$). The IP group showed a higher implantation rate (16.3% vs. 8%, $P = .0005$). Observed effects were independent of clinical or laboratory providers and clinical variables.

Source: http://www.ncbi.nlm.nih.gov/sites/entrez

STUDY CONCLUSION:

This study shows there was a significant higher pregnancy rate in the prayer group as compared to the non prayer group.

YOUR CONCLUSION:

You'll have to decide for yourself whether you want to add prayer to your IVF routine. It does seem though that prayer can't hurt and it just might help.

11. DONOR CYCLE

Sept. 27, 2001

The results were good for donor—fsh at 10 and E2 40 something. It's still hurry up and wait time. She's supposed to start her period the 2nd week in Oct. and from there around 6 weeks to retrieval—so I figure last week in Nov. In the meantime I'm enjoying not being stabbed with needles, and the stress of each appointment. I'm getting a lot of work done on the house and my writing.

I'm also caught up in the IVF bulletin board online— particularly the donor egg section, and find myself spending some time there each day. I cry when one of the women gets a negative beta and feel so happy when someone is pregnant. It's been truly nice to connect with others going through the same thing—some of us may get together in Oct. for lunch.

I had a dream that our donor bailed on us. I don't see this as a sign that that's going to happen but it does show me that there is underlying stress in waiting. My husband, too, shows signs of stress so even though we're getting a physical break from the IVF plunge it still lurks in our minds.

Oct. 8, 2001

Took the first BCP pill today so once more, we're back in the saddle. I'm trying to feel calmer this time and more confident. Must be thoughts of those younger eggs. Sometime this week the donor will have her new patient appointment and then we should be getting the schedule.

Oct. 12, 2001

In about a week I'll be having the ART meeting so then we'll know the dates. Donor is in today or Monday for her new patient appointment.

Last night I had a dream that 3 days post retrieval they did the transfer and they put in 12! I was horrified. And then they told me I had to come back in 2 more days for a 5 day transfer to put more in. Eek! They said not to worry, that it was experimental…I'm glad I woke up.

Oct. 15, 2001

Friday I got a call from the clinic—the old, "Please hold for Dr. X." Of course, I assumed it had to be bad news. Those calls are never good news. The first thing he said was that he'd just given our donor her exam and she's "too good to be true. She's smart as a whip." He had nothing but good things to say about her. As it turned out there wasn't any bad news. She has lots of prefollicles and he said he'd start her on the pill.

There have been so many bumps on the IVF road that to hear all these good things about our donor made me almost as happy as if he'd called to say I was pregnant. So now, I'm moving into that space of enthusiasm and recognizing that we're getting close—only about 5 weeks away from retrieval I think. Because our odds are so high with donor eggs I find myself assuming this is going to work. I surely hope I'm not gravely disappointed. Is it possible that this will be a VERY Merry Xmas? Hot diggity dog.

Oct. 24, 2001

Well, egg retrieval is scheduled for Nov. 26th with transfer on the 29th or Dec. 1st. I begin Lupron on Halloween and we have a scan on the 30th. Here we go!

Oct. 26, 2001

Yesterday the wackiest miracle occurred. I was out walking, feeling rather pissy actually, and I was in a self pitying head down mode thinking about what if this cycle doesn't work. Now, because the odds are so much higher with donor eggs I don't think that too often but for some reason I was really feeling that. I almost stopped walking—"Oh my god, what if this doesn't work?" Just then I looked up and there on the sidewalk in front of me was something pink. I picked it up and low and behold, it was a tiny baby outfit! I laughed out loud. A sign? The humor, timing of it was just too funny and it immediately snapped me out of that negative mode. I continued on my walk, watching for some mother with a stroller to ask if she'd dropped it but saw no one. So, I've started my baby clothes collection. If we only have boys, well I'll give it away. But I consider it a magic onesie.

As we approach this new cycle my body is definitely stressed. Sleep is harder—I find myself lying awake. Very unlike me. And, I've got lots of little itching reactions to something. I feel a bit of ease knowing I don't have to go through stims this time. Yesterday I bought a book titled, "She's having a baby and I'm having a nervous breakdown." I also bought this beautiful card for our egg lady and am thinking about poems for her…I think about her often right now, knowing she'll start injections on the 4th…I wonder what she's thinking now, how she's feeling in all this.

I've been bleeding on and off since last week. Guess my body's a bit screwed up since they started me on pills on the 21st day of my cycle. I'm feeling draggy and more tired than a few weeks ago.

The ladies on the IVF board where I post are great—lots of amusement in a very difficult situation.

The egg retrieval is scheduled for Nov. 26th—right after my brothers leave since they're coming out for Thanksgiving. That should be an interesting week. I think I'll be happy for the distraction at that point. I'm not writing as much as I want or would like. Not sure why. Just, I don't know, seems not as important as this. I'm doing some more work on the garden—trying to make the path more kid friendly and all.

Oct. 31, 2001

Halloween and the first full moon in 46 years—spooky. A good day to start Lupron I say. So in a few hours the injection fun begins.

The appointment went fine yesterday. No cysts—lining around a 6. I never paid much attention to lining before but now of course since it's all I really have to worry about, I am worrying (even though I always have had a good lining).

I thought I wasn't as stressed about the appointments this time since there is less my body has to do. And I was fine all yesterday morning but as we headed down there I realized I was entering that IVF brain cloud space. I'd forgotten, I really had, how disconcerting it all was. Dr. B was hurried but maintaining his dry sense of humor. We picked up all the meds that had been delivered to their office—including the IVIG—intravenous immunoglobulin. I kind of freaked out when I opened the box and the first thing that fell out was an injector for adrenalin in case of anaphylactic shock. Great. Has me a little worried—doesn't everything these days? But, my husband is going to call my Dad later today to set up time for him to do the IV— probably next week.

Today I spent considerable time investigating the numerology of the names we're considering for the kids. Right now at the top of the list is—Nova Ann, Astra King, Rigel William, and Asher King. Still investigating....I know, you don't have to say anything.

I'm weary today. Woke up last night around midnight because of an earthquake. That guy I'm married to slept right through it. Then I couldn't find anything on the news about it because all they're talking about these days is the anthrax threat and terrorism. All of it makes me want to take a nap.

Nov. 2, 2001

Well, this is the 3rd day of Lupron. I was so traumatized by injections in my stomach before—all those calls to family and friends about how hard it was. Well, I guess that seems the least of it now. This time it seems no big deal. Of course, we haven't gotten to the gnarly shots yet—the ones with oil in the big needles. So these first days, until the 12th when I start more injections, will seem relatively easy. Only one shot a day, small needle.

A forty-week pregnancy is calculated retro to your last period—or in IVF case, about 2 weeks before retrieval. That means my first day of pregnancy is in 10 days. Nov. 12. Isn't that strange? I think I'll have to celebrate that day....

Nov. 10, 2001

Well, I've hit that lupron low feeling—thinking that pregnancy is never going to happen for me. I feel as if I'm not really living, but just waiting to see if this works. The black period I would call this. My energy is depleted and I tire easily—some headaches. Yuck.

Tuesday we went up to Dad's house so he could give me my IVIG. I was scared about possible side effects—allergic, allergy. It was actually fun having Dad do it. It took a couple hours and the first half went fine (we had 3 bottles to go through) but then I had this very weird feeling and we had to stop for awhile—run a little glucose etc. When we started I was nervous but everything was fine. I was so relieved when it was over. Now, I hope it does some good.

Nov. 14, 2001

So, on Mon. the 12th I go traipsing in to the hospital to get my blood test. Then I head on over to the RE's but they were way behind so I ended up having to wait a couple hours for my appt. Dr B. puts in the choochie cam and the first thing he says is "Why didn't you have this abnormality removed?" He's talking about the fibroid I have—external, anterior. I said he'd never suggested it. After a pelvic and looking more closely and measuring it he said never mind, sorry to raise false panic. It's far from the lining and my lining has always looked terrific so don't worry about it. Right, like I won't be thinking about that now! The good news, no cysts, and blood tests came back fine so on Mon. night I lowered lupron, started on heparin and Estrace (injection). The Estrace is only every 3 days and even though I don't feel good yet I do feel better than before I started on it. I know the more I get in my system the better I'll feel. I go back again Mon. for blood test again and to look at lining. My donor should be starting stims tomorrow.

My belly is already all black and blue and quite sore. I bruise so easily anyway and the heparin...ouch. The Estrace is in oil and has to be done IM—big needle but at least it's not another belly shot.

I'm feeling very unattractive these days—the lupron seems to bloat the belly out or something and with the bruises, well, you can imagine, not too sexy.

Only 12 more days to egg retrieval. Yikes! It's suddenly coming up...glad family will be here next week to keep me occupied.

Nov. 24, 2001

Got a call on the 16th—yippee! The donor has 16 follicles. Way cool. Quite a different experience than me trying for my own eggs.

On the 19th I went in for a blood test and lining check—a little thin so he raised my Estrace injection a little and I had to go back on Wed. again. This time my lining is at the magic 8B stage—triple pattern, 8mm thick, which is exactly what he wants to see (maybe it was the red wine I had Tues. night). So, I come home to play with my family, here for Thanksgiving week and we wait to hear about the donor's 11/23 appointment. Everything is go—so retrieval is on Mon.

It's the strangest thing—all the waiting and waiting, time seems to go by so slowly. And now, as it gets this close, time is zipping by, though I'm sure it'll slow down again during the two-week wait while we're waiting for the results.

My stomach is so bruised and sore and I'm pretty pissy. I feel a little edge of panic starting, fear, excitement, don't really know what to do with myself. My skin has become super sensitive and the shots seem to be hurting more. Maybe too much violation…I can't believe how hard this is emotionally. I met a woman, who was also giving blood last week, and then saw her in the waiting room at Dr. B's, and we had a nice talk. She commented that she's a really strong woman but this IVF is kicking her butt. I agree. It's very humbling and difficult and no one can know all the emotional and physical violations save the woman herself. It shows though, how strong the drive is for despite all this we go on, toward our ultimate goal of child.

Husband is sick, I'm getting sick, no surprise I guess.

Nov. 26, 2001

Yippee! They retrieved 21 eggs from our donor. I hope she is really happy with herself right now, cause I sure am. This is so so different than struggling to get one paltry egg from my own ancient follicles. Tomorrow we get a fertilization report. My God, it's almost here.

We started the dreaded PIO (progesterone) shot last night. It's so thick it takes a long time to go in but so far I'm not having a reaction which is good.

What a ride.

Nov. 26, 2001

Holy Schlamoly -16 of the eggs were mature and out of those 14 fertilized with ICSI. Amazing. Looks as if we'll be going to 5 day blast transfer which will be on Sat. This is still so surreal. I have the couch/bed all made up downstairs for my down time. I keep expecting something bad to happen—as if I've been conditioned now from my previous cycles. But I am very hopeful that this will work, I know the odds are in our favor. These last days are going by so fast…my butt is sore—both sides. Last night we had to do Estrace and Pio—one in each cheek. Not too fun. But we've never been this far before so I am pretty happy about that.

Nov. 28, 2001

Well, looks like we're going to blastocyst—5 day old embryos. As of today we have 1-6 cell grade 1, 8-4 cell (right where they should be on day 2) grade 1, 1- 3 cell grade 1, 1- 2 cell grade 1, and 5- 2 cell, grade 2. Statistically we can expect to lose a percentage of these by day 5 but this way they'll be able to choose the best to transfer back in.

I'm feeling really weird but could be all the drugs in my body. Started Medrol today, and doxycycline a bit early since I have a sore throat/cold. Wow, this is really happening this time. I'm stunned. I think I need to go lie down.

12. INTERMISSION: PICKING AN EGG DONOR

or can you be the mother of a super-human race?

If you're ever in the position of selecting someone to be your egg donor you may find some interesting emotional issues arise. What, you must ask yourself, are the things that you need to consider?

For starters, do you select an egg donor who is as much like you as possible?

or...Do you decide to improve upon yourself? Maybe someone with fuller thicker hair? Or blue eyes rather than hazel? How can you judge intelligence from a written form and some poorly-taken photographs?

It's an odd feeling going through a stack of potential donor applications and scrutinizing them as if they were prime horses you were going to breed. It's an experience that puts you face to face with the best of your humanity, and the worst. You may have to deal with some of your prejudices…

In my case I found there was one donor who could offer something that was only a remote dream – she was Jewish. And I, having had a life-long love affair with Jewish men, suddenly saw the possibility of having "Jewish" children. Wow. Awesome. She was beautiful, tall (something I'm not) and…whoa. Hold on. Typos in her essay. Not just one but several. And try as I might I couldn't get past that. I simply could not embrace poor-spelling eggs. Geez. How nitpicky is that? (In my defense I am a writer so words are ultra important to me).

The irony is, of course, that with genetics so much is a crap shoot anyway. You can enhance your odds, perhaps, but there are no guarantees. So what then, in the end, is truly important when you choose an egg donor?

Well, I went for someone with a lot more pigment in their skin since we live in Southern California and my pale skin is forever getting burned – and she was athletic during her school years while I was that unfortunate child who was forever being picked last for a team. She didn't look like me at all, but did bear a striking resemblance to one of my nieces. But really, when I read about her, her passions and reasons for wanting to be a donor (for someone she would never meet), I picked an amazing woman who I think, had I ever met, I would like to be friends with.

13. PREGNANT

Dec. 5, 2001

Here I am, 3 wonderful embryos at home in my womb.
When we drove up Sat. we were greeted by the IVF
coordinator who said we had fabulous news waiting for us—
the embies were looking really good. We had the, do we put
back 2 or 3 discussion, and decided on 3. As they prepared
me for the procedure, including letting me take 2 Valium, my
husband and friend got to dress in scrubs. They put me in
stirrups, reclined position, and Dr. B cleaned my cervix etc.
Up on the tv monitor we could see when they put our
embryos into the petri dish—in another room with a
microscope over it fed to the monitor—two close together
and a third a little separate. When Dr. B was ready he yelled
load, and then they sucked up the embryos into a long thin
tube which was then brought to our room, and he inserted
that through my cervix and injected the embryos.

I stayed in that position for about 20 minutes then they
rolled me into recovery where I stayed still for another hour

and a half. I came home to 3 days of bed rest. My friend was here to cater to me so I only got up to pee, I even slept downstairs at night so I didn't have to climb the stairs. I'm taking it all very seriously.

Tues. I had a shower—finally! And have resumed very quiet but normal activities. I've felt pretty lousy, lots of cramping and such, until this morning which was a bit better. Now we wait—blood test in about 10 days. I can hardly believe it—right now there are 3 little ones inside me…how weird is this?

Today I start vaginal suppositories…oh boy.

Dec. 6, , 2001

All I can say about vaginal suppositories is that they're like a party in my vagina no one cleaned up from. Enough said.

So, I'm feeling pretty good, a bit more energy, even did a little plant trimming in the yard though I'm trying not to bend and twist at all. I'm supposed to be on light normal activity—whatever that is. Part of me is anxious of course for my blood test next week but the big part of me is in no hurry because as long as no one (no test) tells me I'm not pregnant then I can imagine and believe I am and for now I don't want that feeling taken away. Not that I have no hope but this thing is so big, so huge, and I've never been really pregnant before so I have no basis of comparison—can't really picture it. That's hard. However, I have done pretty much what can be done—great lining, wonderful embryos, resting properly, etc. I really want to be excited and positive but I want this so much and I'm afraid...other people seem so much more positive and I rely on them.

The time is going by quickly—in 2 days it will have already been a week. Can you believe it?

Dec. 9, 2001

Starting Fri. afternoon I began getting harsh cramps. Yesterday I spent almost all day on the couch. Today, they're still here. I have no idea whether this is a good thing or a bad thing—but it's certainly something. My nipples are a little sore now. Can I be having all these signs and not be pregnant? I may break down and do a pregnancy test tomorrow...it's so difficult when all you can do is wait and over analyze every little twinge (or big twinge as the case may be). I've never had so much attention on my uterus and abdomen. It's so difficult to describe how I feel right now— excited, scared, worried—it's so wonderful to have the IVF connection bulletin board to go to where I know women are going through the same things, the 2 week waiting period, adjusting to the concept of donor eggs. All the aches and pains and worries are shared and you know that you're not the only one cramping, or crying, or wondering. Time for another Tylenol.

Pregnant at last!
Dec. 10, 2001

OMG! I took a pregnancy test this morning and it was positive! I can't believe it—Starting about 2 days ago, other than the cramping, I started spotting (brown, not fresh blood), and yesterday around 3:30 p.m. I was so ravenously hungry. Hubby went out for Chinese but by the time he came home I didn't feel so hungry anymore. Then last night after we went to bed I got so hungry again I knew I absolutely couldn't sleep unless I ate something. For the very first time in my life I actually got out of bed to go get food. After drinking a protein shake I was able to sleep. Until I woke up around 5 a.m. absolutely starving again. I was unprepared for this king of hunger—I'm calling it primal ravenosity. It's a hunger so intense that it overrides anything else.

Thank you great Mother, thank you. It's still sinking in…called family. When I told my younger brother he said, "Excellent." Something about that made me start to cry…So, we made it to this point. How cool is this?

Dec. 13, 2001

Tomorrow is confirming blood test—what a variety of pregnancy symptoms. Today I'm dizzy and the last two days I've been so so very tired. Right after I wake up I feel like I could go back to sleep again. The hunger seems a little diminished though I can't wait to eat or I feel weak very quickly. Lots of weird tugs and pulls in abdomen and my boobs, well, burning, itching, aching—very sensitive. I had a moment of glee today—it might be starting to sink in. Yesterday I took more hpt tests—to see if the line had gotten darker, it had, on same type I took Mon. Then I took another brand just because seeing those two lines form feels as if I've won the lottery. I wrapped one with ribbon and put it on our Christmas tree.

Now, the question is, how many little darlings are in there? Is it more than one? Inquiring minds want to know—many feel all three took. They are supposed to be able to tell us how many with blood test but I know that's not full proof by any means.

Writing this has worn me out…time to rest.

Dec. 15, 2001

Well, yesterday's blood test confirmed the pregnancy. With a beta number of 1385 there's a good chance we have twins in there. It's getting more and more real and I'm so excited about this. Sometimes I feel such happiness I think I could burst…trying to eat enough.

Did I tell you, I'M PREGNANT!

Dec. 17, 2001

Today is our 3rd anniversary. How did we celebrate? We went to Costco and bought some baby clothes. Fun. T-I-R-E-D is the operative word for me these days. I can't believe Christmas is nearly here I've done little decorating and no shopping…we're sending out blast pics instead of presents. I'm so happy to be here.

Dec. 18, 2001

Today I hit a bit of panic as I'm beginning to realize how very different my life is going to be. I don't want to not have that change but it scares me. I always wondered what it felt like to be pregnant and it's such an interesting sensation to realize, hey, there are babies inside me! Often I feel manic joy, other times only tiredness and fear. I'm looking forward to really showing, to feeling first movement, etc. The hunger comes and goes and I mostly feel pressure and fullness in my abdomen. My weight is fluctuating a lot—I was trying to get a baseline weight, good luck on that. I find that I get up and eat, do my shots etc. then check my email and go to my IVF site, and by then I'm already ready for a nap so I lie down for a bit until it's time to eat a snack. Around noon I have to do another suppository (the first one, prometrium, being upon wakening in the morning) which is the messy one (combo progesterone and estrogen). So I usually eat lunch first, then read or rest or watch TV while it absorbs for about 45 minutes. After that I may or may not take a walk, do a little gardening, do nothing except relax, until 3 when I like to watch Oprah. After that, a shower, trying to decide what sounds good for dinner and then most evenings at this point I watch TV. I love the mindless entertainment. More shots, another suppository. Pregnancy post IVF is a lifestyle.

I wish I had a bit more energy but figure if I get one thing done a day I'm doing well. I know if I had to be getting dressed and going to work for someone I'd do it, but since I don't have to I can completely indulge my body in its whims. Whether this is good or bad, I don't know.

I guess I'm going to have to buy a new bra soon as the underwire is getting pretty darn uncomfortable on my current ones. So there you have it, my simple, early pregnancy schedule. Today I'm technically 4 weeks and 6 days into pregnancy.

Dec. 20, 2001

We went in for first ultrasound which revealed—yikes! That all 3 have implanted. However one was much smaller than the other two and educated guess was that it would not make it.

Starting in the afternoon, perhaps seeing them on the screen made it real for my body, I became pretty nauseated.

Dec. 25, 2001

So nauseated we don't go anywhere. Merry Christmas.

Dec. 26, 2001

I had a gush of blood and called doc. I was told to stop heparin and aspirin, and go on bedrest and to come in on the 27th to check.

Dec. 27, 2001

We were sure it had been the 3rd one eliminating itself but ultrasound showed was still there—and though it was bigger than it had been, it was still smaller than the other two. It's possible we saw the heartbeats of the other 2—pretty sure we did but there is lots of pulsating tissue there. Anyway, we go back on the 3rd to see again. So, jury is still out on whether we'll be having 2 or 3 but looks like 2 is more likely.

Dec. 30, 2001

Nearly the new year. Well, I didn't realize how difficult these first weeks would be. I thought because we worked so hard to get pregnant that I'd be nothing but happy. And I am happy but physically—yowza. This is all written in retrospect since I've been really nauseated and on bedrest after bleeding episode...

Now, this nausea thing. Anyone who said eat a couple saltines in the morning really helps I don't think ever had morning (noon and night) sickness. One thing is already very clear to me, when you're pregnant you become your pregnancy. I'm not just Karen being pregnant, I am all the things that I feel, good and bad. I haven't really bonded to this pregnancy yet—it's a process and hard since we don't really know how many etc. And the fatigue. The books say you may have fatigue. What they don't say is you'll feel like you're being constantly sucked at by a black hole of sleepiness, as if you've suddenly contracted some exotic sleeping disease. I didn't expect these first weeks to be so hard. Surprise! Well, one day at a time.

Jan. 2, 2002

A new year has begun. I spent almost all of New Year's day on the couch watching a Twilight Zone marathon…though I did get out for a short walk late in the day. I've been taking a half pill of promethazine for the nausea and that seems to take the edge off though I still find that lying down is the least offensive thing I can do for my body. Today, we're just past 7 weeks…I'm starting to bloat out quite a bit in the stomach, much more in the evening. Can only wear my loosest pants and sweat pants are a big hit with me.

Jan. 5, 2002

Well, ultrasound on the 3rd showed that the 3rd baby has caught up and has heartbeat! However, one of the other 2 which had a heartbeat a week ago, didn't seem to have one this week. So we still don't know how many babies! It would be nice to know and settle in to it but I know sooner or later we'll find out…

I'm trying an electrical wristband for nausea—and seems to be working pretty well so haven't had a pill today. Had moments of almost feeling myself. I actually turned on the garden fountain today.

Many many emotional thoughts but will write of them later—summation, no time to waste, non true things are not worth time.

Jan. 8, 2002

Well, this wrist band seems to really be helping the nausea which has made life oh so much better. I'm anxious about ultrasound on Thurs. This is so hard—no control over anything…we never really do anyway but at least we have the illusion sometimes. Not even a wisp of illusion on this…just riding each day is all I can do.

14. PREGNANCY LOST

Jan. 11, 2002

My heart is breaking—I just can't believe this bad news. The scan yesterday showed no heartbeats. They sent us to the hospital for another scan with more sensitive equipment and that confirmed the worst. It also confirmed a surprise—that there is a 4th baby in there. One of the sacs has 2 identical twins. That makes this all the sadder for me. Now we wait until Mon. to do a final scan and if (as they suspect) that again shows no CV activity then we'll schedule a suction so they can analyze the tissue.

My God, why is this happening? We've seen the little heartbeats and now to have them stop. I go between crying and denial. This just can't be so. I pray, and have everyone praying for a miracle on Mon—maybe that 4th one will come through? It's a miracle that it's even there at all, and full size, when we didn't even see it before. Please please please, let there be at least one heartbeat on Mon. that stays around.

How can this be? Everything seemed to be going so well. The doctor is surprised and flummoxed.

I feel so vulnerable, and at such a loss. The signs were all good—and saying that this was going to happen. Then bam, this. My eyes and head hurt from crying. Damn it! This is not fair. What am I going to do?

Is there still hope? I know the doctors don't think so.

Miracle time.

Warning: pregnancy loss mentioned

Jan. 19, 2002

This is the most awful thing that has ever happened to me. I lost my babies. A final scan last Mon. confirmed that they had indeed stopped developing so we scheduled a suction for Tues. The procedure lasted longer than I expected—he'd said it was a little complex because there were three sacs and my uterus was enlarged enough so it would take a bit longer. I had trouble post anesthetic with nausea and by the time they had given me medicine for that it turned into an all day procedure. But worst of all is the emotional pain.

This is the worst, deep grief of my life. So fundamental to being a woman. Losing a child is indescribable deep black helplessness. I know it could have been worse. I could have been further along, the children could have been born then died…I feel so terrible for all mothers who have suffered such a loss. It seems impossible that anyone can really survive it, yet somehow we do.

Each night I dream my babies are still alive, and then each morning I wake up and reality comes crashing in, the pain is fresh and new, and I cry again. I seem to cry at odd times, often. I crave affection from hubby —it's as if my body is afraid and needs the reassurance that it is still there and alive. There are really no words to describe how this feels. I will never be the same. I will always mourn the loss of these four children. Everything aches, my bones, my heart, my uterus, my soul. And my body still looks and feels pregnant which is a cruel mockery. Part of me is still in denial—this can't possibly have really happened. When will I wake up? Soon I hope. This is a nightmare I never want to have again.

I'm so afraid to try again—to use those frozen embryos. I'll be terrified every step of the way—particularly if we get no answers as to why this could have happened. We had more blood drawn for further antibody testing. The fetal tissue was sent out for analysis which might give us some answers, though unlikely. And then there's the possibility that my fibroid, even though it's on the outside of my uterus could have compromised the bloodflow although there are no stats backing up that my type of fibroid can have that kind of effect. Though if we find no other reason at all, I suppose we'll have to take that step to have it removed before using the frozen embryos.

Right now, all I expect from myself is to try and get up each day and put clothes on. Beyond that, anything else is a plus. Time will help heal, but will not take what has happened away.

I still long for my children. And I want these four back. Why has this happened?

Jan. 24, 2002

Bone weary. Grief does that.

My husband and I went away for a few days and it was great reconnecting with him. My birthday was on the 21st and that was a really sad day since I couldn't help but think of what might have been. But, we got through it and ate lots of good food. I'm beginning to realize that I'm going to have good moments, and not good moments. Just like any portion of live. These emotions may be more extreme or amplified compared to what I'm used to but it still boils down to good and bad moments. I'm trying, one step at a time.

Jan. 30, 2002

Saw the RE yesterday. No tissue results yet. This is what we know. My immune system is more active than we thought. Also, I have that external fibroid that is good sized and Dr. B feels pretty strongly we should remove it. So, I have a procedure scheduled for end of Feb. for him to look at it and we hope he can remove it with scope and laser so I don't have to have an incision. If he can remove it then I have a 6 week recovery. If he has to do it by incision, I have to take lupron first and that'll take another 6 weeks. This cycle, before using frozen embies, I'll have to use prednisone (yuck) starting at about 6 weeks prior to transfer. I'll also have to do about 3 rounds of IVIG instead of just the one we did this time. So, all the drugs we used before, plus some. We're looking at at June/July cycle. Seems so far away. But I know my body needs to recover. I still look pregnant, and I'm up 20 pounds, and of course I still have emotional healing to do. I do feel better after yesterday knowing that they did find some things that we can 'fix.' It doesn't mean of course that these are the things that caused the problem or that this guarantees success, but at least we can be proactive. But, we have a plan of sorts now. We do want to use up the frozen embryos, it's so relatively inexpensive there's no reason not to. But I'm not happy about yet another procedure, or two, and additional drugs, especially prednisone as I know how weird/crappy that makes me feel. And on top of lupron…I hope no one sticks a gun in my hand.

I'm still sad and grieving and soon will do some sort of closure ceremony to help me release energy etc. and try to move on. But in my heart, there are now, and will always be, my four little angels.

Feb. 13, 2002

Finally yesterday we got the fetal tissue results—of the cells they analyzed all were boys, and all were genetically normal. This is good because it means that our frozen embryos are all probably just fine.

The hard part is knowing they were boys makes them so much more real to me and now it's not just the pregnancy I lost, it's my boys. Doubled with knowing it was most likely my immune system—it's hard not to think of my body as a baby-killing machine. That may sound harsh but when you can't succeed at the most basic of biological female functions it's hard not to judge oneself.

I cried today for the loss of my (our) boys. Mostly I'm getting less sad emotionally but still there are days…and I don't want to harp on it with either my husband or others. I know even with tragedies people get tired of hearing about it. Thank goodness I have the link and support of women on the internet—women who've gone through what I've gone through and they are always there for me. Several I've even connected with on a personal level. One thing this journey has done is hugely increased my respect for women. I see a strength in me I didn't know was there and I also see the great strength in the women around me, particularly those that are high lighted for me right now, those going through infertility. We forget I think, that what we're actually dealing with is a medical condition and not something we did wrong. Over and over I've seen women comment, does this mean I'm not meant to have children? Does God think I'd be a bad mother? The answers, as I see them, are no and no. Just because someone gets cancer it does not mean they are no longer meant to be alive. It's a journey, like IVF. Some people with cancer will die. Some women with infertility will not end up with children. But many will. I do believe there is something in the journey that is teaching us something we want to learn or we wouldn't be going through it. Granted, it's a hard way to learn a lesson. Infertility strikes at the heart of womanhood (and manhood) for who are we if we can not procreate? Isn't that, in a biological sense, or single biggest drive, need, responsibility? It's one thing to choose not to have children. It's another to desire them and be unable to produce them. There is something in the basicness of it that makes us feel it's our right to be able to produce when we want to, just as it's our right to eat when we're hungry. And when we can't succeed there's a huge amount of frustration, anger, disappointment that goes along with that.

I love my life. Yet, now, at this time in my life, I'd also love to have children, to have that experience of raising eager young minds and getting to know them as people. It will add a new depth to my life that can not be felt with any other thing. For so many years I did not want children and feel I lived a good and full life. I've lived hard, experienced much. Yet somehow I know that the intangible quality of fulfillment will increase tenfold with the addition of children to our lives. I only hope I get that opportunity.

Despite the pain and awful sadness of my loss, I also feel a peace. Somehow it has fueled my beliefs that things happen for reasons, even when we can't understand those reasons. I trust that the miscarriage was a 'good' thing in the cosmic sense and I trust that we will use those frozen tots and be successful. Yes, I will feel new fears I didn't feel before. But I believe in the message that the movie, "Defending Your Life" portrays. We are here to face our fears, and go through them. When we lose it's not because we failed, but because we never tried, because we let fear deter us. I see people all over living lives of fear, afraid to really let go and LIVE. But isn't that why we're here? We will never be totally fearless, it's what we do with that that matters.

So, I will face this fear, and go through the actions that will take me into the heart of it, and I will pray and hope that this time when we come out the end of this long dark infertility tunnel, we will have our children here with us, sharing their lives with ours.

15. INTERMISSION:
THE LADY'S GUIDE TO IVF LINGO

Blastocyst

The goal you'll have for your embryos because success rates are higher. For healthy embryos the blastocyst stage usually happens at around 5 days post fertilization.

Cooter Cam

That penis shaped ultrasound device which is inserted into the vagina to view the uterus and monitor egg development. For a time, your life will revolve around this "penis" and not that other one (much to the dismay of your male partner, if you have one).

Embies, Embryos

Your babies. At least that's how you'll come to think of them. After sperm and egg are united and start to split they grow for several days – those are embryos.

FET – Frozen Embryo Transfer

Miracles. When embryos that have been frozen are transferred into your uterus.

ICSI

Stands for Intracytoplasmic Sperm Injection. What? Basically a microscopic procedure to assist fertilization of the egg by directly injecting the sperm into the egg cytoplasm.

Totsicles - Frokids – Frozen Embryos

Your frozen babies. Embryos that are frozen prior to implantation in you but to you they'll already be your babies.

3-Day Transfer

When embryos are transferred into you 3 days after they are fertilized.

5-Day Transfer

When embryos are transferred into you 5 days (blastocyst stage) after they are fertilized.

Dreaded 2-Week Wait

That period of time where your life is suspended, you're afraid to breath, and you'll suddenly become superstitious. The 2-week period between embryos being put into you, and the time when you can have a blood test to check for pregnancy.

16. BETWEEN CYCLES: SURGERY

Feb. 22, 2002

Got away for a few days—business trip up to Monterey.

Yesterday we went in for pre-op appt. and I ended up getting really angry. Rage actually. Don't know all the reasons why. I was hoping the surgery on Tuesday would end with the removal of my fibroid but it sounds as if that's unlikely. He's going to do a biopsy and also search for endometriosis. If he can lasso the fibroid and take it out, he will. If not, we'll have to wait 6 more weeks, use lupron to shrink the fibroid, then take it out with myomectomy which is much like a C-section. I don't want to go through more damn procedures. When is enough enough? And I'm worried about the odds of a frozen embryo transfer - going through all this and then the prednisone on top of everything else…will it all lead to naught?

I just feel so frustrated and overwhelmed. Drowning. And it's coming out as rage at everything.

Feb. 25, 2002

Well, surgery is tomorrow. Some of the rage has passed only to be replaced by tears. I find myself crying even when I don't feel consciously sad. Don't know what that means exactly.

We saw the movie Dragonfly yesterday and it had a section where one character (a nun) is talking about different levels of consciousness and anesthesia. It made me think that perhaps when under I can experiment with different levels of consciousness. I'd love to come back with memory of what I've done, where I've been. And even though I've thought a bit about death I do want to come back from this.

Though I've accepted that this next step is part of the process I'm still not excited about doing it. I think too, it's a definite statement that we will be cycling again and that brings up the fear of facing the potential loss again.

I want to be pregnant again.

I fear being pregnant again and losing babies again.

This next time will work.

March 4, 2002

I'm healing pretty nicely though still popping pain pills. My left ovary area hurts. Dr. B gave us a nice home video of the beginning of the surgery. Sadly, they didn't get the fibroid but he did get a lot of endometriosis and adhesions. So that was all good however I have to go through another surgery probably in May. A myomectomy. What a major drag.

When I woke up from the anesthesia I remembered being in a good place but couldn't remember where exactly. I didn't have any nausea this time.

In this IVF journey sometimes I think it's the waiting that's the hardest part. When in cycle at least I feel like I'm being proactive and I suppose that gives some illusion of control while during the wait I feel like I'm just drifting. I try and function and pretend I'm a normal functioning human being but on the inside all I'm thinking about is baby/s. I see how IVF becomes a thing unto itself and I don't want to lose sight of why we're doing this. As I said in the beginning, I don't want to make this a way of life. I'll give it this year, and then if I feel like it hasn't worked we'll need to move on. I can only sense how hard that would be…of course, if the upcoming FET works then by the end of this year we'll be well along in our pregnancy.

Please God, let this FET work and let the pregnancy stay.

I keep telling myself to keep this all in perspective. My neighbor and friend was diagnosed with breast cancer and she just had a mastectomy a few days ago. In about a month she'll have to start chemo. Whenever I start to really feel sorry for myself I think of her and am ashamed. But that doesn't stop the sadness and wishing and wanting. I pray and hope that by the end of this year she is fine, and I'm pregnant. That's not asking too much is it?

March 11, 2002

This has been a very bad weekend. Dr. B's office called at the end of last week to discuss the pill/lupron schedule to shrink the fibroid. This is lupron Depot which is once per month, time release. I was happy for a day that we were getting going on next phase but then the depression really hit. I guess starting up lupron on Tues. has brought it all back to me—the pain of loss, the terrible mood swings while on these drugs…and it's not even as if this lupron is the mark of a cycle. I'm also really mad at the husband because I tried to engage him this weekend—emotionally. I told him I was sad and all these issues have come back up again—even how many totsicles to put back in. He couldn't seem to get into an emotional space at all and it really struck me hard. After all, part of why I'm doing this is his genetic link. I've already given up on mine and would be quite willing to adopt. Anyway, feeling very alone with all this. Thank goodness for some of the ladies from IVF connections, particularly the ones I've gotten to 'know' a little bit. It's the saving grace.

We go back to Dr. B tomorrow for our post op and for him to do a scan to check for cysts. Seems kind of silly since he just had his hands in my guts and if there were cysts he would have taken them out then. Oh well. He has a conservative nature but maybe that's what makes him so good.

The skin glue is finally peeling off and the scars from last surgery are minimal. My belly button, site of one incision, is still a bit sore (as are my innards) and I noticed once the glue was gone that it looks a little different than it did. Does this mean, I am reborn?

March 13, 2002

What a wreck I've been this week. When we went to Dr. B's—can you believe it, a cyst on my right ovary! Unbelievable. I was in such a space that I really challenged Dr. B. He told me we'd rescan that we can't start lupron with a cyst of this size. I said why not? I'm not worried about egg quality. I said I heard what he was saying that it wasn't a good idea but could we start anyway. He said that would be malpractice. Guess he felt pretty serious about this. I had a list of questions, and tried to not get too stuck on yet another delay. (I keep asking myself, do I want to do this fast, or do it right?). Anyway, he ended up saying that I didn't realize how personally he and his staff take the results they get. I said in fact, that I had some idea because I saw him. What I meant by that was, that after the scan when the hearts had stopped, and we went back in just to be sure, it was like his whole body had collapsed in upon itself. I appreciate that this is not just about making money for him. It some small way it makes me feel less alone.

I know I'm supposed to let go of this schedule I have in my head and to go more with the flow but it's so difficult when your whole life is wrapped up in IVF. Even though I'm in between it's out there looming so I don't seem able to really have 'other life' and then once you're on drugs well you're not really yourself anyway. So, there is great internal pressure to push forward as rapidly as possible to either get to 'life with kids' or try and create new life without kids.

All this has led to depression for me. I feel I don't have any stamina left, emotionally, or otherwise. This last year has basically beaten me to a pulp. I guess a feeling of hopelessness is the sensation. Something very foreign to me.

March 20, 2002

Vernal Equinox today. As of Mon. the cyst was still there. I go again on the 25th to check one more time. If it's no smaller we'll consider aspiration. I'm actually going through a phase of feeling a little calmer about the wait. What else can I do? It seems expressing my frustration to Dr. B. really helped me to not carry it around. I know this is a good lesson in acceptance. I'm trying.

Though I'm still sad, my energy is returning somewhat and I'm able to get excited about the garden and house again. We just replaced the entertainment center in the master bedroom. It was a soulless piece of pressed wood. Now it's pine which we stained black. Seems we kind of have an Asian Safari theme going in the master bedroom sitting area. Guess I'll be focusing on these simple things for awhile. Chop wood; carry water.

Grief is the darndest thing. It kind of hangs around for a long time and sometimes you forget it's there. Then, at an odd moment when the blue in the sky is just right, it sneaks out and gnaws at your heart and there is nothing you can do but give into it.

I was talking to someone the other day and they commented that if there are too many obstacles in the way that it must mean that I shouldn't be doing this. I used to think that too about things but I don't know. Perhaps because I'm in the middle of it. Perhaps because any dream worth having is a dream worth pursuing. As my dear friend pointed out, literature and entertainment is filled with stories about someone who faced impossible odds to climb that mountain. Where would we be if they had given up?

March 28, 2002

We went in on the 25th to find that the cyst was not only still there but larger. Time to aspirate. We got a call later that they could get us in the next morning for surgery. And I had gotten approval to have the procedure done without a general anesthetic. I hate coming out of that. Then of course I was a little worried that maybe it would hurt too much. But by the morning of the 26th I knew it was the right thing for me. I still didn't eat or drink just in case. When the anesthesiologist came in she didn't believe me that Dr. B had approved the procedure with no general. She said he always has his patients out. Well after she spoke with him she came back to speak with me. She was worried that if I moved at the wrong time I could perforate a bowel or something. But I was certain, and very calm. I had no fear at all, my body was not even afraid. Finally we agreed upon just a mild IV sedation but I would be fully awake. It was kind of weird being awake for all the vaginal prep etc. Once Dr. B came in he started right in, we talked about books, he told me to take a deep breath and let it out slowly, probably as much to distract me as anything. There was pain but by the time it registered it wasn't so bad at all and then we had to wait for the cyst to drain. It was a big one and the liquid from it ended up filling an entire urine specimen cup. He showed me the liquid…and then it was done. I could have walked out of the operating room—still on the happy drugs. Well, after a very brief recovery we went down to the office to get the lupron shot—before another cyst could grow.

So, all in one day, cyst gone, started on lupron depot, and I got to have surgery without all that time recovering from the anesthetic. It felt very right to be going outside the normal medical construct for this and it worked out so great all the way around. Dr. B also told my husband that he was reasonably certain he could get the fibroid out with scope surgery after it shrinks which would be great because it would mean I don't have to have a full myomectomy. Much less recovery time. I felt as if a great deal of energy had cleared up on Tues. Perhaps he sucked out all the bad stuff with the liquid.

April 2, 2002

Saw Dr. B again yesterday. All is AOK. I'm about to finish bcp's which I've had to overlap with the lupron. The lupron is giving me terrible insomnia so I got something to help me sleep as I'm sure I can't stand another 5 weeks of not sleeping like this. Now I'm focusing on an upcoming vacation and trying to divide the time left before I can be pregnant again into cycles. Vacation, then only 1 week until I see Dr. B again at which point we'll probably schedule the fibroid surgery, then recovery time, start prednisone, and the cycle begins. It seems to make the time shorter when I think in phases.

In addition to the insomnia, my energy level is terribly low—boy do I miss estrogen! I really appreciate how good it makes my body feel when I'm on lupron and my system gets shut down. Pretty awful feeling actually.

April 3, 2002

Saw Michael J. Fox on Oprah today. His story serves to remind how very lucky and blessed I am. My father also has Parkinson's.

I would like to know Michael J. Fox personnally.

Oprah, too, for that matter.

A good reminder on a day I needed it. I did a ceremony for my babies this morning. I cried. It was good and healing.

April 30, 2002

The last day of the month. The effects of the lupron this month have not been too terrible. Bad headaches but any pain killer does the trick. My energy is much better. Had a great vacation up in Vancouver and I came back with a new attitude. In fact, I feel great for no apparent reason. We finally scheduled the (I hope) last surgery to remove the fibroid. This is to happen on the 28th of May. Then, from what I understand, I have to recoup for about 6 weeks and I also have to be on prednisone for about a month before we could transfer. So, probably August before I'm pregnant again.

This has been a strange, sometimes awful, sometimes interesting, sometimes good, journey. My entire attitude about women has changed. Before I had little respect for my own sex and now I see us as much stronger than I would have imagined. I've met some incredible women because of my IVF journey. From the Internet boards I post on there is this link to women. While on my Canada trip I met two of the women. It's so strange to think that though we'd never met in body here we were, chatting away as old friends. The intimate link comes partly, I think, from the nature of infertility. The discussions on the board are very personal and deal with something that is a fundamental drive for the entire human species. How much more basic than that can it get? These are women that I would most likely have gone my entire life without ever meeting. Something entirely wonderful from something so bad. There is also my now close cyber friend who lives on the East coast who also had a pregnancy loss. With her I was able to express lots of my pain and loss after a point when others would probably tire of hearing about it. Thank the Goddess for her.

And then there's my new more local friend who I've met a couple times. She just had another negative Beta. I am so sad for her. It's amazing how much I care about these women and what happens to them.

And the one I'd never met until a week ago but whom I'd spoken to on the phone a number of times. She and her husband decided to adopt and within a few months their little girl was born. For them, that journey was quick and really reinforced that that was the decision that was right for them.

And so, we continue on. Each in their own way trying to get to parenthood. Most of us will succeed, some will move onto getting on with their lives without children.

Would I trade infertility away if it meant I'd never have met these women? That's tough but I'd have to say no. I wouldn't want things to be any different than they are. That's today at least. And today is a good day.

May 14, 2002

The lupron has given me terrible insomnia and having to use sleeping pills to sleep is getting old. I try to not use them and then I truly can't sleep. I guess I just try and muddle through until the effects wear off which I hope won't be too many weeks past the fibroid surgery—which is only 2 weeks away now. In some ways it seems like forever getting here. In other ways, seems like no time at all.

Two days ago was Mother's Day. Hubby took me out for a wonderful brunch but I confess the sadness was lurking all day. If my pregnancy had lasted I would have been 6 months along…I try not to think of that. The good side. It's very hot out and I would have been pretty miserable—these hot flashes are bad enough with the recent heat wave.

I repainted my entire office, as I couldn't stand the way it was before. It just wasn't me anymore. Now it's a dark sultry deep spice color. And I painted part of the bathroom too since it just wasn't cutting it in all white. I'm using tiger pattern and leopard as accent…I have been getting a lot done as of late. My energy is much more than I ever could have imagined while on lupron and in general I've been in an excellent mood.

Many failures on the board lately…It's hard to see so many women who truly want children to have it remain still out of reach….

Had lunch on Sat. with one of my new IVF friends. She's ready to move on to donor eggs so I got to rehash everything and I remembered stuff that has long been out of my mind. It's so strange to realize that it hasn't even been a year yet that we started on this donor egg path.

May 22, 2002

Well, the good times are over. Hit an emotional brick wall a few days ago.

Yesterday we met with Dr. Brody for preop. It sounds as if there is a greater possibility than I thought that he might have to do a full myomectomy—which means at least an overnight stay in the hospital. That scares me. I hoping of course that he can still do it all by scope. Even though the incisions will have to be a bit bigger than the previous scope surgery it is surely the way to go. I know he's a great surgeon but I'm still afraid. In part, not only because of the surgery itself, but what it marks. This means that after I recover I will be cycling again and all that that entails. Hence the fear.

I leave for a conference tomorrow and won't be back until the night before the surgery so next time I make notes here it will be post fibroid surgery. Let's hope that he's able to do the entire thing without having to make a major incision.

At least this marks the end of my surgeries. I hope.

I really hope.

17. INTERMISSION:
INFERTILITY RESOURCES

Finding support is key. Locate a forum you like, meet other women, share, and be together on your journey. There are tons of sites out there. Here are some to get you started.

<u>IVE Connections</u> : support, forums, articles, information and more

> http://www.ivfconnections.com/

<u>IVF Forum</u>

http://www.ivfconnections.com/forums/register.php

Facts, Resources, Experts

http://www.ivfconnections.com/forums/content.php?308-Links-to-IVF-Facts-   Resources-Experts-Support

Alternative Treatments

http://www.ivfconnections.com/forums/content.php?348-Alternative-   Treatments

Fertile Thoughts: support, forums, articles, information and more

http://www.fertilethoughts.com/

Forum

http://www.fertilethoughts.com/forums/infertility/

Blogs

http://www.fertilethoughts.com/forums/blogs/

Infertility Myths and Facts

http://www.fertilethoughts.com/index.php?option=com_content&task=view&i   d=15&Itemid=18

18. POST FIBROID SURGERY

June 7, 2002

It's been 10 days since my surgery. As I write this I realize that for you, the reader, from the previous line to this line only a few seconds have passed but for me days and days...the surgery turned out well though it was a long procedure. He did not have to do a full open myomectomy and he gave us a video of the entire procedure. Tedious work to take out the fibroid through the incisions...had to open up the skin around it and then laser it out along the skin and then cut the entire fibroid out. Then he ground it up with something he calls a morselater—like a mini meat grinder. Anyway, there was little blood loss and no perforation of the uterus. That said, it was way more painful afterward than I could have imagined. They had me on morphine for a bit and even though the surgery started at around 10 I didn't even start to wake up until 4. I couldn't believe how much it hurt. I finally forced myself to begin waking up and opted for an oral percocet instead of more morphine because I wanted to get home that day. When they finally moved me to the post op area and removed my catheter I felt like I had to pee so I had to get up and use a commode…wow! Ouch. The ride home was long and each bump in the freeway was awful but was glad to get home to my own bed.

Thank goodness we did this while my husband was on a week vacation because I really needed his help. It's been a long slow recovery. I finally got off vicodin a few days ago and though I'm still quite tender (there are 3 incisions plus the navel) I feel better for not being doped up.

And so, we heal.

June 13, 2002

We had our post op on the 11th. All looks fine and we talked about what next. Something I didn't really know was that even though there was no perforation of the uterus now that it's been operated on, it is not as strong as before. So, Dr. B. talked about selective reduction and that even if I am pregnant with 3 I should probably reduce to 2. I have to do more research on the odds of a problem…but at this point we're thinking about putting 3 embryos back in if they thaw well and look good. If they don't look great we might put in more, should we have that choice. It's possible, I know, that not all will survive the thaw.

We asked about the hot flashes which I still have from the lupron effects and he said let's just put you on the pill and they'll go right away. And they have. Yeah! One less thing to be battling in my body right now. I don't feel pain anymore but do feel discomfort and am very aware of my incisions and abdominal area. Sometimes it's worse than other times. Sadly, my back is unhappy with all the resting-recouping-lounging and it decided to cramp up on Sun. so now I'm dealing with that too. I'm just kind of a mess from my navel down.

So, the plans are... I do this cycle of pills and after my period I'll go in for a hysteroscopy so he can check to make sure all the stuff he's done hasn't caused any new problems. Then, I'll start cycling. My best guess is 2-3rd week in Aug. for FET. I was so hoping to be pregnant before Aug. 20 which was my due date. Wouldn't it be weird if the transfer ended up being on that day? Anyway, I have mixed feelings about getting going because of my fear of losing another pregnancy. How does one forge ahead and not feel that? I know I can't control these things and we've done/are doing all that we can do to help the pregnancy stay. What more could we do? But, I'm afraid. I guess all I can do is one day at a time and hope that this time we will bring out baby/s home in good health and that at long last we can experience being parents.

19. WE CYCLE AGAIN

June 24, 2002

Anger. I am angry that I have to start all over again. It's like my 'enforced break' was a honeymoon period emotionally because all I had to deal with was my body healing. Now, here we go again, ground zero. I know in reality it's not quite that but emotionally it is. My original due date was Aug. 20 and as we approach that I feel disoriented as if somehow I stepped off the right path that would lead to the birth of my children and now I find myself here on this, someone else's, path. I'm proud and pleased with the women I've met through this but still, how did I ever get from, I'll never try…to here? A vast fertility wasteland of shots and emotions and pain and yes, some joy, but mostly struggles. On my favorite board, IVF connections, they just put up a veterans board, and it's so sad to see how many women are there after years of struggle and round after round of IVF. The drive is strong, the ability to say enough and let go, difficult at best. I feel like we've all gotten in this boat that's heading toward a waterfall and we can't get off.

I'm sure I'm no pleasure to live with right now. On the physical front, I am feeling a bit better. Actually took a walk today. I was like an old lady huffing around the block. And to think I used to run marathons. Wow.

And on we go.

June 25, 2002

Well, got the rough schedule today and as I thought the transfer will be around Aug. 20-22. I actually feel in a bit better mood now that I can actually look at the schedule. I almost feel a tinge of excitement. Official first date of cycle start is July 9.

Hotter than blazes here today. Time to watch Dr. Phil on Oprah.

July 8, 2002

It's amazing how the IVF roller coaster gets going and immediately I become a control freak and things that I should take in stride become much more important. My period started on the 5th and since I'd thought it would be a couple days sooner than that I started getting all stressed about it. How sad is that? Things happen in their time. I know this. I believe this. Yet I had to have a long talk with myself about easing down the path instead of trying to manhandle everything—particularly the things that are out of my control.

July 10, 2002

Spiritual freedom. Pursuing that which scares you to death. Last year I dealt a lot with the idea that you lose your freedom when you have children. A concept that all of society has bought into. For me, having avoided children, taking on this fear and having children is the only thing that will truly set me free. I got that today in a conversation with one of my spiritual friends. I now see fear as a signpost pointing toward that which will liberate you. For once fears are walked through and you see that you survive, you are more free than before. Universal fear is death. But body death truly sets the spirit free. Here though I speak of spiritual freedom, rather than spirit freedom. Spiritual freedom comes from pursuit of soul desires and working on those things which have burdened us for lifetimes. At least, that's what I believe. Spiritual freedom is something you can take forward with you into the next life, the next step so that you don't start again within the confines of that particular fear. I see now, how very important this children thing is for me. This is why I have pursued this even through all the hell and pain and loss. In the big sense there is nothing more important than spiritual freedom. That above all else must be the cosmic goal of each life. So I see now. I can not give up, must not give up. I want to be free. Ironic that something I spent so many years running from is that which I need most. So, fear, conscious or not, makes us want to run when what we really need to do is turn and face it and try and understand whether there is a piece of freedom for us nestled within the fear.

The new cycle started yesterday. Transfer will be Aug. 23. I am another step closer to my own true spiritual freedom. This is what I tell myself – this kind of thinking helps me survive.

July 18, 2002

Well, we're off for a vacation in a couple days. While there, I start lupron and prednisone…sigh. Here we go again. My back has been all out of whack and I'm sure it's fear and emotions all balled up into the small of my back…but forward we go. Once again I'm getting excited about possibility…

Have I mentioned the singing turtle we have? Remind me to tell you about it sometime. A kid's toy that seems to go off on its own these days…only 1 song a day. I think my children are here playing.

July 21, 2002

The scan on Friday did not, of course, go entirely smoothly. Another cyst. Geez. Dr. B wanted to hold off a week and I didn't because my previous experience tells me that we could sit on this thing for weeks. The entire thing is complicated by the fact that we leave today for vacation and Dr. B. leaves the day after we get back. So, despite his recommendation to not start lupron, I'm going to start. He did kind of say it was up to me. He also said that if they rescanned in a week and the cyst was the same or smaller I could start then. But I have to say, psychologically I just can't see waiting. I know we may be slowed because of this anyway but there is a chance it will just go away on its own and then we're off and rolling. Taking the delay now makes the delay certain whereas going ahead with lupron means there's a chance we go ahead as scheduled.

I recognized just how little resistance I have left for snafus. I didn't feel the panic I have before, that clawing desperate feeling that I have to go forward, rather a very calm gut level, that says we should go forward. So, we are. So, the day we fly back we have to rush right from the airport down to San Diego for an appt. to see what things look like then. What we'll do if it's bigger I don't know. I'll cross that bridge if need be.

I spoke with one of my new IVF buds yesterday and I have to say, only another IVF person can talk about a cyst for an hour. But I found it helpful to cover all the ins and outs, to make sure I'm not being pig-headed stupid about this, and to get another opinion from someone who has been there. I so want things to move forward quickly and well even though I have my fears. Standing still does nothing but make me feel stuck in the fear.

So, in 2 days I'll start the lupron and also the prednisone which, I hope, will have the grand side affect of helping my back which has been really hurting.

I've been burying myself in house projects and recognize that that's keeping me sane. For me right now it is very true that idle hands…and of course there is the side benefit that the children will be able to live in a lovely decorated home should they care about such things. The older I get the more important keeping a good house is to me. And the daughter becomes her mother.

Aug. 4, 2002

Well, all is well. When we got back from our vacation, a great "do nothing" sort of week, we had to drive the 1.5 plus hours right to the Dr.s office for scan. And the cyst was gone! Yeah yeah yeah. Gone. I'm so glad I started lupron. So we continue on. Tomorrow I go for first E2 count, and start estrogen which will be nice as I'm starting into minor hot flashes and insomnia at this point. I'm also starting lovenox which is a low molecular weight heparin so I only have to inject once per day instead of twice. It's also supposed to bruise less which would be nice considering I still have faint bruises on my stomach from 7 months ago.

I'm feeling optimistic these days. I'm still afraid but have a sort of peace inside me. I don't know what that means but I'll take it. I have been keeping very busy so I don't obsess too much about everything and the house is the better for it so at least there is that. I've been building a fireplace mantel which has been a challenge considering I've never plastered before, or tiled, or several of the things that I had to do to create this unique mantel.

Today I'm going to lunch with 3 other women from the IVF board. One is a woman I have met before so that'll be nice. Another I haven't met yet. The other, one of the original women I met in San Diego is at long last pregnant and I think this was her 5th IVF round. I'm so happy for her. Another of the women I met back then, who'd tried round after round, finally switched to donor eggs and she is nearly past her first trimester with twins.

I can't believe how long it's been since I was pregnant and miscarried. But I have to say, in the last couple weeks, I'm looking forward to being pregnant again.

Aug. 10, 2002

I went all wiggy yesterday. Today looking back I feel like some scary demon woman possessed me. Couldn't make decisions etc. I think the stress of the cycle is starting to fray me a bit around the edges. Not much I can do except stay busy and keep my mind on the moment at hand.

My stomach is horribly bruised from the lovenox injections and whoever said that it doesn't sting as much as heparin was wrong or lying outright.

Hot hot hot here today. I'm sweating just typing this.

Aug. 13, 2002

Well, thank the goddess, my back is finally better. Yesterday I did the IVIG at Dr. B's office. After having the vein blown in my right hand we got it going in my left arm. All in all it went pretty quickly and smoothly but frankly, I still feel punk. More tired than I should. Perhaps it was the stress. Who knows. It could be the prednisone too. So many different drugs in my system. Anyway, the good news is, my lining is ready to go. Already triple pattern and 10mm. My E2 was 171. So, now we hurry up and wait some more. Only 9 more days…

I find myself trying to stay mentally distracted so I don't start to obsess about the upcoming cycle. Yeah, good luck with that. We've done all we can do. I keep telling myself that. Mostly I feel mentally pretty good.

Today I had a long discussion with my new IVF buddy "S." We talked about how many embryos to put back in. I've long been hovering at 3 and she was questioning that—thankfully, to make me really think. I know Dr. B said that I probably shouldn't try and carry 3 since my uterus has been operated on but I need to do more research and gather more information. I'm afraid to "only" put in 2, not sure why. I admit to being influenced by the fact that I'd love to have twins. It's so hard to know and ultimately, no one can say what will happen. What to base the decision on? I'll think about it more for now though I'm still leaning toward 3…

I can't help wondering, where will I be 2 months from now? Will I be well into my pregnancy? I surely with all my heart and soul hope so…

Aug. 15, 2002

I feel very punk today. And the days are getting a bit longer…8 days to go but then that's only the beginning. Faith faith faith. I know. I can't tell you how important my new friends are becoming to me. Other women who have been through some of the same hell I have and who totally get the picture. I am doing better with the shots this time. Not letting it affect me as much. Though between my bruised stomach and my scars from surgery I'm not looking all that sexy these days. Or at least not feeling that way. Yesterday I felt great. Today, like shit. I'd forgotten the ups ands downs. Hormonal, stress related. Who knows. But it is what it is and I know this is such a small part of the big picture. Sometimes I have to marvel at the struggles we humans go through and yet we go on, keep ticking away. Not always with a happy smile but nevertheless, we keep going. That in itself is amazing. At times like these I think of people who really inspire me—who have, are dealing with immense physical obstacles—Christopher Reeves is the number one person I think of and how, despite his paralysis, he still is contributing to and changing the world in a good way. I can't think of him and not get teary eyed. Then there is Michael J. Fox, with his Parkinson's, whom I also think of a lot. Perhaps because my dad has Parkinson's it means even more to me. In reading Michael's book I'm amazed at his attitude. I try and be positive and all in all I do well. But there are those days like today, when it's just damn hard.

For many people I know, this has been a difficult year. I wish and pray that for all who are struggling toward something they dearly want, that they get what they want and need.

Aug. 19, 2002

Final scan done this morning. A little trauma and drama. The triple layer patter on my lining was harder to see and this was a concern—until we found out after Dr. B took a look at the pictures that this is how it looks at this point. The fact that I had the triple layer (B pattern) means I'm good to go—10 mm thickness. We got all our final prescriptions.

I am having anxiety and having some trouble sleeping. I try hard to focus on the good things and not the possible "what ifs" but some days it's more difficult than others. I thank my lucky stars that I have good friends like I do. That makes the journey so much better.

Only 4 more sleeps to go, as we say on the board. So soon so soon. Remember Karen, what will be... will be.

Time for some wine.

20. EMBRYO TRANSFER AND THE DREADED TWO WEEK WAIT

Aug. 22, 2002

Amazingly, my transfer is tomorrow. Less than 24 hours to go. Wow. I painted the hallway this morning - saved it so I could be busy. We just got back from renting 5 videos, and I have the bed made up in my office since I'm not supposed to climb stairs for a couple days. I'll be sleeping in my office — first time since we've moved here.

I'm excited and nervous and scared. I so hope to get pregnant again this time and of course have it last. Please please please universe, make this be the time that leads to me having my healthy baby/s.

Aug. 23, 2002

Today's the day. We leave in about an hour. Amazing. Here already. I'm feeling such a range of emotions — been teary eyed a couple times already...what a day this will be. Next time I write my frokids will be home safe and sound and snug inside me.

Aug. 25, 2002

Well, here I am on bedrest, in my casita so I'm typing this from the bed. The transfer on Fri. went really well. They only had to thaw 3 to get 3 good ones so we still have 2 left should we ever need them. This was such a different experience than the last transfer—which was hushed and reverent. This time my friend S was there with her husband for a procedure they were having. And the transfer was in Dr. B's office instead of the surgery center. So, I stripped from the waist down, sporting my one blue and one pink sock—hubby was wearing the other 2—and got up on the table. They brought in a couple warm blankets for me. Then S popped her head in and took a few pre pictures.

Dr. B came in and seemed a little amazed at all the activity. After S left he got down to business and prepped me. Nothing about it was uncomfortable except that speculum…so, he did all that he had to do and then he let the nurse know he was ready. It's like a team relay—someone holding open each door, and the embryologist comes through, tray in hand (S clapped as it went by). Dr. B did his magic and inserted the little babes—they checked out that none were left and then we were done. I had to lay there for 15 minutes with my legs still in the stirrups and then I could stretch out and had to rest for another hour. During that time, S and her husband came in, K, another woman from the board popped by with her stepgrandson, and we had ourselves a little gabfest. So there we all were, 6 of us in that tiny room with me on valium. The time flew by, as you can imagine. The nurses popped their heads in a few times but could clearly see all was fine. After I could get up, we did a few more pictures and then we took off, me in the reclined front seat.

Came home and stretched out. Will be on bedrest through the weekend but this time since I'm sleeping in the casita I can use the computer.

Now I have to try and not analyze every little sensation. I just went back to my notes from the last transfer to see what the symptoms were and it seems 6 days post transfer I had really bad cramping. We'll see what happens this time. Everyone is so confident that I'll be pregnant again. I hope I can keep my fear at bay for the first weeks. But I feel calm, at least right now, and maybe I can stay that way. Please please please universe, please, let me get through this pregnancy with healthy baby/s. I'm so ready to be a mom.

Aug. 26, 2002

Feeling pretty punk today—is that a good sign? Though I'm up and about now it's more like up for a bit and then down resting for a long while.

The big question, if, and when to do the dreaded evil pee stick test?

I actually ordered 2 little baby outfits today.

Aug. 27, 2002

Feeling very very crabby cranky today. Woke up feeling that way—no apparent reason. Also started those wonderful vaginal suppositories today. Here we go again with hopefully a better ending, or beginning as it may be...I can't remember if I felt cranky like this in the last cycle—I didn't make note of it if I did. I'm also having some nasal congestion and mild cramping off and on.

I took a short walk this morning and that felt good.

Aug. 28, 2002

Very crampy today.

Still a little crabby too.

Aug. 29, 2002

Well, feeling pretty good today—is that good or bad? I feel the hpt test calling me but it's still too soon I think...6 days post transfer. I'm almost halfway to the beta test...trying not to be too anxious.

Aug. 31, 2002

Yesterday I took an hpt—negative. But I didn't totally wig out as it was only day 7 and I didn't do it in the morning...this morning I took an ultra sensitive test and it shows a faint faint 2nd line—you know the kind where if you turn it to the light just right and squint and tilt your head it's there...could it be? Am I pregnant again?

The blood test yesterday showed that my progesterone (about 54) and estrogen (around 800) levels are what they want them to be.

I feel excited—a little reserved until I see a darker line on another test and everything is confirmed by blood test on Fri.

Today, lunch with IVF gals, some whom I haven't seen since I first met them last Oct.—2 have had their babies and I know at least one will be there today. Yeah!

Sept. 2, 2002

Day 10 post transfer. HPT's are all coming out with 2 lines. Having terrible insomnia. Today also started some brown spotting—implantation spotting I'm sure. Lots of uterine pressure and off and on mild cramping. Nothing near as uncomfortable as last time though.

The lunch was great on Sat. Nice to have 2 babies there and catch up with everyone. What long roads we've all walked...afterwards S and I actually went to a sale and I bought some 2 baby outfits...safari style!

My dear friend C tells me I don't need to have fear. I'll try and hold onto that thought when I begin to worry.

Pregnant Again
Sept. 10, 2002

I'm pregnant again! Beta came back lower than I anticipated (it's those expectations that always get us into trouble)—it was 265. Probably means there is only one. I'm thrilled to be pregnant again but find myself grieving for the one or two that didn't implant. So far I don't feel sick but the fatigue is overwhelming. The fact that it's so hot outside doesn't help, no doubt, and I do find the hunger thing is increasing. My body is definitely not my own and that's just fine. There's such an amazing feeling just knowing you're pregnant. Even when I feel bad I feel happy.

The fear comes and goes and mostly I'm trying to stay in the moment for in this moment everything is good. Anytime I'm still pregnant is a good time.

Had a long family weekend this last weekend and it was great to see everyone—a good distraction from obsessing too much.

Now I just have to get through the next few weeks without being too fearful. Just get to see 2 ultrasounds with the heartbeat still looking good and the pattern will be broken.

Sept. 11, 2002

Anniversary day of the terrible tragedy of last year. The baby shows today are showing babies that were born exactly 9 months after 9/11/01. Lots of emotion.

Yesterday and today I'm kind of a draggy girl. Did go for my walk this morning but found I ran out of breath easily. Then I did some computer work for a couple hours and then I just had to lie down on the couch for a while. I'm so grateful that I don't feel sick. I'm so grateful to be pregnant again. This pregnancy feels more integrated than the last one. Don't know quite how to explain it. More a part of me? More natural or something.

Sept. 13, 2002

Fri. the 13th. I woke up this morning with the most amazing feeling—a realization that I'm pregnant. There's something about it. Even if you do nothing else all day you know you're doing something great and wonderful. Life.

I'm trying to keep my fear minimal as I don't want it overriding moments of joy and in this moment everything is good. I did hit a couple days of yuck and called a friend to help me work through it. I have no place to go but forward and really think I'm doing pretty well considering my body doesn't have anything to compare to except my previous sad experience. Spiritually I am happy and feel good and sense that this pregnancy will last and I'll end up with one or two healthy babies. It's just that my body is not so sure. Will have to keep talking to it, telling it each day that all is well.

Shortly I leave for my first appt.—a cervix check. Scan is not until next week…

Sept. 17, 2002

The cervix check was all AOK. Dr. B asked me about all my symptoms and he said everything looked as it should. My bp was up (for me anyway—at 110/80) so I know I am stressed. Each day I wake up and each day I still feel pregnant—pretty symptomatic—cramps (mild to moderate), hunger pains at all hours, a bit of nausea in the last few days but not bad— nipple soreness etc.—and a fullness in my abdominal area— all these things I enjoy because they tell me all is fine inside. We have our first scan in 2 days and will then know more…the women on the board are taking bets on how many and what sex baby/s are. My husband came home yesterday and said he had this strong sense that it's one and it's a boy. I'm trying to just stay open to whatever it/they are…

As each day passes and I still find myself pregnant I think I get a little happier, a little more in the mode that this truly is going to work and I'll get one or two of 'dem babies. I so want to enjoy each moment of this time so try not to focus too much on the next appt. etc. For now all is well and I am content. Life is good.

Sept. 18, 2002

I think I'll call this phase the hunger phase whereas last week would be the fatigue phase. I'm hungry a lot and with almost no nausea it makes me happy. I'm a lucky woman.

Minor bleed (fresh blood) scared the hell out of me. Not more than a couple teaspoons but still, very scary.

Sept. 23, 2002

The ultrasound on the 19th was good. We saw the heartbeat and a baby that's measuring a good week ahead of schedule. There was also a shadow of a 2nd something but looks as if there is only one baby this time. General consensus says it's a boy.

I was very nervous (and my bp reflected my fear) just prior to the actual scan. Each morning when I wake up and there are still symptoms I'm happy about that. This next u/s will be on the same day as the last time we got a good u/s so if we can go one week after that perhaps I can relax a little more…be present in the joy, not the fear.

Breath and surrender.

Sept. 27, 2002

Ultrasound yesterday was great. Can see the armbud forming and also little white lines where bones are starting…and the liquid space where the brain will be. Size is good (13 mm) and the heartbeat looked strong.

Nausea set in a few days ago though this morning isn't too bad. It's also cooler outside which is a relief since it's been hot even at night. Perhaps fall is finally here.

We are now within a few days of when I lost my previous pregnancy so I am anxious to make it through this week and see good things on the u/s next week. It's hard, this uncertainty. But then, that's how it is with children, and life for that matter. Can't control anything other than one's self reactions. Sometimes that stinks.

Keep your fingers crossed that this time we go all the way to healthy baby.

Oct. 3, 2002

Feeling like crud this morning. Part of it stress—u/s later today. But I still feel pregnant so that's good.

I'm finding that it's hard to keep hold of myself while pregnant. Since I must give my body over to the baby for its use, what of me? Already I struggle with holding onto me, the things I want to do, and not giving all of me over to whatever the baby wants and needs. I can see how women get so buried in motherhood and lose themselves as individuals. For a time, it's natural I suppose, as you tend to this helpless tiny creature that relies on you.

So how can one do it, hang onto self, when part of you is the baby? My writing, my career, is very important to me. Yet I find its current importance seemingly diminished in light of my current 'creation.'

Oct. 4, 2002

Yesterday's ultrasound was good. I was very scared—my palms were even sweating. But the little one is doing fine— 21 mm, all curled up, head and body. Since this was the equivalent time frame of that fateful ultrasound last time, I wonder, will I be able to relax more now? Actually, I've been pretty relaxed most of the time. I guess what I mean is, will I stress out this much before each u/s? We'll only have 4 more visits to Dr. B's office. It's been such a part of my life for so long that'll be weird. I'll miss the people.

My symptoms are persistent and that's okay with me. I'm tired a lot again. If I don't eat often the nausea is pretty bad at moments. My heart seems to pound, some dizzy spells but not extreme, gas, and hunger. The slowed digestion is hard on some days but all is all I feel not too shabby for an old pregnant lady.

Oct. 11, 2002

Great ultrasound yesterday! We saw our little one move. It was the coolest thing I've ever seen. He/she's up about 40% in size from last week, has 2 arms and 2 legs...really looking like a baby in there.

We got our babybeat monitor today. Couldn't find the heartbeat but could hear my heartbeat maternal sounds, placental sounds (like wind), some movement sounds...blurp...very noisy in there. This is getting very real.

Oct. 17, 2002

Another great u/s today although our attempts to get it on video failed. Anyway, baby was swimming all around, moving arms and legs etc. Very cool. Development is around

10w3d which is good. We're at 10w4d. Yikes! Hard to believe I'm this far along already though you can tell by looking at my stomach. I'm definitely looking pregnant and my boob growth is, well, it's there. I'm already up one size…and can only really wear sweatpants at this point.

Oct. 24, 2002

We met with the regular OB today. It was weird, being in the waiting room with all those women who got pregnant by having sex. I really like the doc, she's young and vivacious, and seemed very understanding about how hard it was for us to get to where we are. She does not categorize me as high risk and we'll only see her every 4 weeks up until week 30. She moved up my due date to May 11, one day earlier. She did a great scan and pointed out things we hadn't seen before. Fingers, toes, jaw bones. Pretty cool.

Oct. 28, 2002

12 weeks, one day. Nearly to the 2nd trimester. I went down Fri. for appt. at B's office. My friend met me there, as she wanted to see the scan. We did manage to get a video but baby was not cooperative, as he/she wouldn't move around. Guess the little one is already independent. It was interesting to get 2 scans back to back and see the differences in measurement. OB measured baby as 12 weeks at 11w4dy and nurse measured at 11w4d at 11w5d. (the measurement differential was 2mm). Just shows how hard it is to measure that early on.

So, I have one more appt. with Dr. B during week 13. Then I'm cut loose. Yikes! Will see Ob again on 11/22 but won't have scan again until Dec. when we do the level 2 for diagnostics and sex determination. Just like being a regular pregnant woman.

I had my friend take some belly shots of me. When she emailed the pictures to me it was weird because even though I see myself in the mirror it wasn't until looking at the pictures that I could see wow, I really look pregnant. I think I'm big for 12 weeks but hey, it is what it is. My rapid weight gain that occurred during the first 10 weeks seems to have slowed. I'm sure mostly due to the fact that this new phase of nausea is not helped by eating and it's hard to find anything that sounds appealing. So, I'm eating less than I was. I'm also still doing my 30 minutes of walking every day.

I don't think I'm to the point yet where I've really integrated the fact that I'm pregnant. I mean really pregnant. That we're going to have a baby in a little over 6 months.

Am I ready?

Nov. 3, 2002

Today begins the 2nd trimester. Yeah!

Nov. 11, 2002

Well, I feel like I'm getting bigger by the minute. And the magical no more morning sickness in 2nd trimester doesn't seem entirely true for me...but it is better. One of my IVF friends was supposed to have her transfer on Fri. but none of the embies were genetically viable. Very sad news. I feel so bad for her. It does remind me however of how hard we worked to get to this point and to be grateful for where I am, pregnant, and things seem to be going well. No matter how cruddy I feel on some days.

We have our last appt. with Dr. B tomorrow. So hard to believe.

Nov. 12, 2002

So, we graduated from Dr. B's. It was sad and a bit hard actually. My husband said he felt anxiety because it was like we were letting go of our lifeline.

The u/s went well. Good heartbeat, good size—70mm. Dr. B also did a ph test because he said if it's under 4 it indicates an infection which can lead to premature labor. I checked out fine. He told me he wanted me to come back, but we won't be making a weekly trek down there. I know, moving forward, this is all good.

Nov. 13, 2002

Today I feel better. This morning I felt terrific. My waist is really popping out and I feel some pressure/discomfort as everything gets squished and pushed aside. My breasts are still as sore as ever. I'm starting to get excited about possibility...are we really going to have an actual baby?

Wow. That concept is hard to believe really. Such a life-altering event. The other day I was thinking how weird it was that I have 2 heartbeats in my body now. How cool is that?

So, we're getting there, day by day.

I'm scared.

Excited.

I wonder.

21. MY BABY IS BORN

Feb. 28, 2003

Into the third trimester. A friend of mine threw a baby shower for me last weekend. Really interesting mix of my IVF board buddies and my relatives. I've known all along how important the support is that I get from other IVF gals but was reminded again when some of my relations commented on how bonded we ivf ladies are—even those I'd never met in person before. If you have to go through fertility treatments I can't express enough how important it is to have a support group like this.

The last couple months have certainly been the best of the pregnancy. Doing the baby's room (by the way, IT'S A GIRL! And we're going to name her Kaley), feeling the vigorous kicking. It still takes me by surprise to feel her moving. And it seems so strange that there's an actual whole human being inside of me. As my belly gets bigger and bigger it gets harder to deny that this is really happening.

last in the 3rd trimester so he could see me. And he said it's good to breastfeed for 6 months while taking Omega 3 as this will increase baby's IQ by 4 points. And he said the baby should be vaccinated with individual vaccinations to avoid the potential link between autism and the cluster vaccinations. (LA times today had an article saying there is no link though not everyone agrees with the study).

It was a good appointment. They've been such a part of our lives for so long I admit to feeling a little lost knowing

We started birth preparation classes this week. I was surprised when the nurse asked how many were planning on an epidural that I was the only one not to raise my hand. I know most women end up with one but didn't realize that so many go in planning on having one. I've also received the information for hypnobirthing which is a style similar to the mediation I already do. I'm really hoping to use that to stay drug free. But, if I really need them I'll use them and not feel bad about it. I'm trying to view this just as I would training for a marathon. Do what I can to ready my body, my mind, and spirit. The great unknown. I'll try and see this as an adventure.

The whole thing is mind boggling really. How hard it was to get to this point, that we're really where we are...miracle truly.

March 19, 2003

I knew we'd be the oldest people in our child prep classes but at least there is another couple that are 40. Of course, they were lucky enough to get pregnant the old fashioned way. The class is good in that it gives us all the facts of what can, should, may happen. Also, the what could go wrong stuff and about drugs.

I'm just past 32 weeks. I'm tired a lot and am busting at the seams but really, I feel pretty good. I'm enjoying the way my body feels and don't mind the beautiful rounded belly at all—though my feet aren't too thrilled with the weight gain. The last few OB appointments have been routine. Baby is measuring ahead which is good despite the fact that I'm not putting on much weight in this 3rd trimester. I guess that's because I put on so much early on.

Sleeping is a challenge. I have to get up so often to pee I wonder, why don't I just sleep on the toilet? Sometimes in the first hours of going to bed I have to go every 20 minutes.

I so rarely think about the fact that this child was created with donor eggs. No, I haven't forgotten my donor or the wonderful thing she did for us, but it's just that, well, this is my baby. I feel her inside me, kicking and dancing and whatever else she's doing. How could I think otherwise? Sometimes I'll put headphones on my tummy and play classical music for her. The kicking is different than I thought it would be. When it first started it was in isolated spots which is how I thought it would be. Now, when she really gets going the whole uterus moves. I'll miss feeling her inside.

I still can't believe there's a whole smaller person in me. What an amazing concept.

I love the feeling of walking around pregnant. It just feels good all over.

May 13, 2003

On this day, my first child, Kaley was born. Large and healthy, born the day after mother's day.

Hey, did I tell you, I'm a mom now!

22. CONCLUSION, FINAL THOUGHTS

At long last I come to write the end of this particular saga and though my years in the IVF reality game are over, I know that for many it is just beginning. When my daughter was 1 we put in our last 2 frozen embryos and both took so at the ripe old age of 48 I gave birth to twin boys, both over 7 pounds, I'm proud to say. Now, my daughter is 7+ and my boys are 5+ and I can finally say that now I go long periods of time without thinking about how I came to have my children – they are simply and so complicatedly, my wonderful children. Yes, telling them how they were conceived is something we are open about and about the use of donor eggs as well. They love hearing the story about the generous "egg lady" and the doctor who helped make the in such a special way.

The greatest things, other than my children, that came from this IVF journey, are the strong long lasting friendships I've made with some women – women I would never have met if I had not had to go through this. I also developed a

in new admiration for the great strength of women. So, at this point, I can't even say I wished it had never happened. And of course, once you meet your child/ren, you would never trade them (well, except yesterday when one of my boys peed on the couch on purpose) and you know that how you got them is part of who they are. The most important thing you can do for yourself when you're going through IVF is get a support system of women going through the same thing. No one else will be willing to obsess about every little aspect, except another who has been there, or is currently there. There are some dynamite online support systems and I encourage you to check them out.

It takes amazing courage to go through IVF – to want something so much you stick with it until you find your own solution "baby." You can't go through it and not be altered in many ways – some of them wonderful. I hope that hearing this first hand uncensored account through the land of IVF will help you feel just a little less alone when you need it most. We're all here – all the women who came before to this reality game. We are holding your hand in spirit and we all applaud your courage.

ABOUT THE AUTHOR

Karen Daniels has four previously published books including a family book, "Baybo, The Baby About to Be Born," which is a story for families created with in-vitro fertilization and adoption. Karen is an internationally published poet, online content specialist and creativity mentor. Her friends consider her renegade, spiritual, and a bit odd. She lives in Southern California with her three miracle children.

Find Karen at karendaniels.com or on her blog zencopy.com.